CONTENTS

INTRODUCTION

" Birthing babies With the Big O "

A new layer to the of Science of birthing babies.

The status quo. By the time you become pregnant, chances are you have observed many people on TV and in movies having painful, difficult births, complete with screaming, crying and lots of drugs, where an epidural is an expectation rather than a possibility. But what if birth didn't have to be anything like that?

What if you could choose.

What if you could choose pleasure over pain. The potential for orgasmic birth is great. Not just by luck or by an act of faith and prayer, but by volition. By choice of an awakened woman to use her own sexual nature to enhance her experience of child birth. And feel less pain.
Birthing Babies with the Big O Is an intensely open, sensitively crafted, empowering and upbeat, guide to Orgasmic Child birth.

And Yes - It is an actual thing.

This strikingly Intimate guide to fundamentals of orgasmic child birth. Piece by piece covering why, how, who and what is all you need to know. The anatomy of orgasm. How they happen, how to make them happen and all of the spaces in between. The anatomy of the female form, pleasure centres, the physical and chemical trail that binds birthing and orgasms together. Overcoming cultural barriers to feminine empower-ment.
Mind bending perspectives that will show the true connection between birth and arousal, how your body was designed to birth, and that orgasms aren't just for enjoyment but become a whole new layer to the science of birthing babies.

Authored by World Class Personal Empowerment Expert Victoria Whitney and its accompanying Audio programme and Online course You have your entire pregnancy and birthing journey mapped out. Victoria has a successful career working with 1:1 clients and has also worked in the NHS and Health and social care environment for the past 20 years.

In person she has a wealth and calm essence in addition to her wealth of experience the vibrancy and energy she has are unique. Victoria is a Multi Award Winning Personal Empowerment Expert Awarded for Inspiring Human Potential and Coach of the year in the Wouth west of England 3 years consecutively, with 21 years experience having qualified in Hypnotherapy specifically for child birth in 2012 ahead of the birth of her son. Victoria has a fascinating insightful dynamic which she is renowned for making the most complex of ideas appear very simple. "Birthing Babies with the big O " Is a natural progression and accompaniment to "Birthing Babies - The Ultimate guide to a positively Empowered Birth" each have facets the other does not contain and will build together a very powerful foundation for your Birthing Journey and beyond.

Including
1. Introduction (The boring bit)
2. The anatomy of orgasm.
3.The mechanics of the female body - Your Physical body. Orgasm and birth.
4. The science, Mind, body, Birth and Orgasm.
5. Labour.
6. Accepting Female sensuality in birth - Overcoming Social and ecological challenges to Birthing babies with the Big O.
7. Expansion of the prospect of pain relief.

Alongside powerful insights and inspiring motivational perspectives, birthing babies " with the Big O " contains fascinating insights which will turn the beliefs you have about how we birth babies on their head. Bringing a whole new perspective to child birth. To move beyond anecdote to real scientific computations which turn an insane idea, into something you cannot not do. Because it makes sense. Your body was built for it and you will learn how here.

All covered with the warmth and appreciation of how all these can be included in a dignified and empowering way to redefine how women birth. Redefining how women define themselves sexually, and bringing greater satisfaction to life, love and the birthing suite .

Copyright Victoria Whitney © 2026

" We may lay it down That pleasure is a movement, a movement by which the soul as a whole is consciously brought into its natural state of being, and that pain is opposite" Aristoltle

Why does it sound so cosmic. Orgasmic child birth. Of course. Wild. yes. Insane. Most likely, but reading on you will find how the pattern intricately woven by your design makes it not only possible, but potentially one of the greatest solutions of our time in the management of pain in child birth. There are growing bodies of evidence both scientific and anecdotal which suggest that sexual stimulation can diminish pain during child birth therefore avoiding the use of pain relief medication. On a grander scale Awakening of the pleasure sensors through sexual arousal can result in a reduced requirement for pain relief. That is a reduced experience of pain.

This is ground breaking, because the potential is huge across all facets of pain management. Starting at the beginning. Birth. The potential for orgasmic birth is great. Not just by luck or by an act of faith and prayer, but by volition. By choice of an awakened woman to use her own sexual nature to enhance her experience of child birth. And feel less pain. Without shame, embarrassment. Quietly and privately, accepting her own sexuality in a different way to be embraced as it was originally intended.

Orgasmic birth here, goes beyond the anecdotal stories in the media of spontaneous climactic births. Also known as an ecstatic birth, orgasmic birth is essentially the idea that some people may be able to experience an orgasm, during childbirth. This orgasm could occur spontaneously. Women who can by, positioning, and luck experience an orgasm as baby passes through the birth canal touching pleasure sensors, presses directly into the G- spot as it turns the corner and crowns. Include the perfect balance hormones oxytocin, of love and the circumstances align to make that possible that is spontaneous orgasmic birth. It is possible. But that is different.

You can't plan for that. Nor can you learn it or even very well control it. However. The alternative perspective.
Is that a woman can use arousal, to influence the biochemical load, during child birth, in synergy with the natural hormone release during birth to magnify the sensation of pleasure and overcome the sense of pain by literally flushing the senses with the directly opposite force. Pleasure.

This is explained in detail, because it is a systematic mirror of the natural flow of labour, where each change chemically functionally is matched with an equal and synergistic purpose when arousal and labour are combined. With the aim of making birth not just pleasurable but to use the bodies own formation and system to engage a flow of pain relief secondary though mirrored to the flow of labour which merges with each phase and step and by flooding pain sensors with an increase in natural hormones, makes pain less prominent. Reduces stress, brings calm and good health.

The difference is. You are choosing to do this with volition. Birthing babies includes the importance of the 3 c's being calm, confident adn in control. You are not even just choosing to make arousal and sexual pleasure part of your pain management routine in labour. You are engaging the chemical and hormone release to enhance every stage of labour and make the fourth C climax one that brings great pleasure, but also great birth.
It is plausible, the next few chapters will show you how, why and bring the pieces together that make this make sense. So it is not just another hipster movement. It is so much more, like a fundamental scientific revelation. That supports all women, to birth more comfortably.

The idea of a pleasurable birth is something that birth doula Debra Pascali-Bonaro — who directed a documentary on the subject in 2009 — has been advocating for a long time. In fact, on her website, she calls it "every woman's human right."
Regarding spontaneous Orgasmic birth evidence of this is predominantly anecdotal. There limited scientific research on the phenomenon. That it could occur in about 0.3 percent of vaginal births spontaneously.
without effort.
The anecdotal discoveries support the notion in theory, when the position of baby passing through the birth canal such that the angle and exact pressure on the g spot on its jour-

ney through the birth canal it is possible, to cause an orgasm to cause a surge of intense pleasure so great that it eases the sensation of the final moments of labour and turns them instead into a surge of ecstasy. More so it is plausible that the birth canal was designed this way to affect the inclusion of the intensity of orgasmic pain relieving sensation as it passes through the birth canal into the most physically demanding moments of childbirth.

At the exact time when you need it most, when the cervix is fully dilated and the perinium, and vaginal walls are at their most stretched to fill those muscular tracks with a release of the pleasure hormones, which relax, engorge, at the very moment when the body needs it the most.

With the chemical and physical synergy that occurs when you orgasm being perfectly timed to with the most intense moments of child birth .

Where the greatest sense of relaxation and opening is intended to flood the sense with pleasure sensations. At specifically the times when birth would be most uncomfortable. For relaxation of the musculature that is most called to stretch and move while it's contracting at specifically the times when it's at it's greatest pressure. To bring waves of chemical and hormonal relief to the places which need them most to make birth more effective, more efficient and more comfortable.

Dr. Christiane Northrup, a board-certified OB-GYN and author of "Women's Bodies, Women's Wisdom" and "Mother-Daughter Wisdom," said orgasms during labor are caused by basic science.

"When the baby's coming down the birth canal, remember, it's going through the exact same positions as something going in, the penis going into the vagina, to cause an orgasm," Northrup said. "And labor itself is associated with a huge hormonal change in the body, way more prolactin, way more oxytocin, way more beta-endorphins -- these are the molecules of ecstasy."

The reasoning that the baby is moving through the same parts of your body that are involved in sexual pleasure, preludes the pleasure centres being an active part of child birth. If you can begin to wrap your mind around it, as you move through this text you will begin to appreciate this is an asset. The anecdotal reports surround the spontaneous pleasure are many in number however, there is growing evidence that making love, and organismic pleasure increases the chemical responses in the body to active rewire the experience of pain.

Just imagine, being able to control your level of pain. Advancements in child birth has been life changing in its evolutional progression over most recent years. This is the next level of enhancement of a woman to be pain free and in turn make her birth the ultimate pleasure.
There are so many reasons why you should. So many reasons. When you combine it with the potential to actually directly manipulate, the chemical balance to pleasure rather than pain the two will make child birth something so new and revolutionary. The strangest dichotomy is that uncovering this knowledge might appear revolutionary but its a return to our origins. What our body was originally designed and built to do.

The fears, the stressors, can be overcome with hypnotherapy for child birth and guided relaxation. By building confidence and to really apply these techniques, to really get the reason, the science the synergy and to accept the difference between sex, and arousal in the birthing process. To accept your ability to be aroused in these circumstances and know that it is within the purity of childbirth that this is so. To be comfortable with this not as just an idea but an actual workable and real life solution to enhance your experience of birth another level. As a natural progression, and to experience the sense of arousal making pain relief, pain literally turning into climactic pleasure. With the active intention of guiding and manipulating, controlling the chemical responses and transitions through birth to be complementary and to progress labour in efficiency.

Why you could. Why you can, why you should, and how you can, are all here.

Of course, there are barriers to whether you can, whether you would. But reading this it is possible to reason and overcome those barriers because the strengths the advantages the possible benefits outweigh the reasons by far. And you can still honour many of the existing barriers whilst still experiencing orgasmic birth by choice. You have the potential to make childbirth more efficient, so you are less tired, put less strain on your body, on your nervous system. To preserve your energy, and to birth more comfortably. By using your bodies own natural resources to their greatest advantage.

The possibilities for pain management, Sexual arousal giving rise to pain relief, are commonly recognised. You can google articles for orgasms and pain relief. It is widely evidenced. But is it widely believed and used.
Here you are actively learning how, with growing bodies of evidence to reveal the possibilities. In this context specifically in Birthing babies.

Beyond that you can take it where you want. I'm a great believer in once you learn first principles and have a solid grounding in knowledge, which has been proved and tested then you can expand it, and play with it, to take it to new areas. To make the possibilities spread and become great new opportunities and solutions.

How to know if you're a good candidate for it.

You can not plan for a spontaneous orgasmic birth but you can learn how to make one. This is what is written and believed, but when it is not a spontaneous unplanned gift delivered to the few but a skill and a choice that is the potential for the many. It's different and that is the reality of the now. The main barrier to over come is whether you believe you can, whether fear, embarrassment or ego will prevent you. Or if you can overcome the social preconceptions and assert very gently and quietly a principle that the woman as you're designed in your perfection is able. As you read on and discover more about the body the womb, the cycles of labour and the role of the clitoris. Here I will guide you to change pre conceptions and open the possibility of that. Not just maybe you can, that you certainly will.

Whether you can achieve arousal and orgasm is without question a yes.

During your experience of labour even in the most intense moments it is possible to re route the pain sensations. Becoming sensations of discomfort and then climactic sensations of pleasure. Working through the text you can imagine how the experience of orgasm is perfectly suited to complement child birth and enhance it. To the point where it is natural to ask the question was this how we were designed to birth in the very beginning.

Naturally there will be exceptions to the rule, those who anatomically physically cannot birth baby naturally and this is something we accept. Birthing babies will always include a percentage of interventions a percentage of caesarean, forceps, ventuese delivery and a percentage of episiotomy. But it doesn't have to be expected, and you can do everything within you to make it possible that intervention is not required. In cases where it is you are forgiving accepting and experience a sense of accomplishment no matter what.

The aim is unnecessary intervention, instances where Intervention could have been avoided. These are reduced to the very bare minimum. By increasing each woman's ability to birth with a sense of calm, confidence, control and climax. Imagine if we were to, Replace the chemical numbness with mental re assignment of the pain receptors and a climax, excitement that actively supports the progression of labour by mirroring the muscle pre programmed experiences and instinctive reflexes, strengthened them and made them feel good. That is something, much more than a nothing. Imagine the difference, when you birth with joy rather than fear, and birth with pleasure. There are so many potentials, faster healing in the body, less stressors the impact could be so much more beneficial to both you and baby. So read on as the conceptual realisation of the potential will become an actual possible reality and even an experience. Seeing as the one percent chance of your baby moving through the birth canal at the exact angle required, to touch the g spot and produce a spontaneous orgasm. Is so finite, too finite to rely upon, that's chance, now you can have choice to be more than a one percent and actively learn to reduce pain in birth by turning it into pleasure.

So you know, What an orgasmic birth is, that they are possible, not just spontaneously but when you actually believe that they are possible, and that you can choose to. That you can use your body's own cycles to and chemical trail to overcome discomfort in labour. You are beginning to wrap your head around the possibility that it is an actual real life possibility more so than a joke, or a laughable notion. Something that has the potential to change peoples lives.

CHAPTER ONE

INTRODUCTION
(the boring bit)

"Life is tough enough without having someone kick you from the inside." – Rita Rudner

This is a valuable guide to using simple and effective techniques to expand the possibilities for what labour and birth can be. The aim. Make Childbirth as comfortable as possible, and make comfortable birth accessible to as many women as possible. To build confidence in women to birth their babies as they intend. And experience significantly less pain. By bringing to life hidden education which demonstrates the latencies of the female body and how they can possibly find new purpose in the place of child birth.

For the modern woman who is "everything". " Birthing babies with the big O " Includes missing insights which give you the reader the knowledge and power to birth their baby with confidence. Things we do not get taught at school. To redefine their preconceived ideas about childbirth, their bodies. What is possible and acceptable in child birth because the science begins to teach you that perhaps the way women were organically designed in their origination holds the keys for our evolution. The big O is potentially one of the most controversial, yet ground breaking possibilities. Which will in time be normalised and become just as hypnotherapy for child birth has in recent years, not just acceptable but the norm. The go to. For women who birth. It's dignified and personal and something that women can begin to cherish. And accept absorb and allow themselves to own.

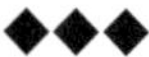

It begins. You are pregnant. You might be celebrating or in overwhelm, but the feels are real. It's Happening. And it's ok, even if it doesn't feel like it. There is few words that can encapsulate the feeling of pregnancy for the first time as every one's journey is different and everyone's journey, is unique. The journey can be defined by something more though. The journey can be defined by your choice to explore the possibilities of a natural birth. A birth with less pain. A birth where you are at one with yourself and at one with baby. A connected birth.

This book will take you through the insights and experience of Doctors and theorists and bring approaches to you that will provide the support, the sustenance and the emotional direction to birth baby without fear, the physical ways to birth baby with less pain.
To build clarity calm confidence so you are in control in your childbirth experience. You can choose to use your bodies great strengths latent until now, to bring about a revolutionary birth, and to redefine your sense as a woman.

You can make your birthing journey an empowered one. Not the huge overwhelming power, but the silent inner stance that is educated refined and beautiful. That is power embodied within you as a woman who can birth her baby with confidence. To embrace your body, the intricacies. The unknowns and explore. For you as a woman to precede and to predict your life moving forwards including, and evolving the education of the other facets of childbirth. The untold truths that make you more empowered than you could know.

The word empowered is overused now, so much it's a branding tool that has been milked of its sentiment of truth and real meaning, however, in this instance it means Awakened, reestablished, educated, competent, able to choose with great strength, feminine, and beautiful, strong and able. Someone who has the ability to move her world, and does so as she chooses. In essence it is within you in its finest form and comes from a silent intention and in context a silent promise to intend and determine your pregnancy and birthing journey. To intend a calm composure and to intend that you are educated, and to experience the joy of the journey, of the evolution moving forward. That is to predict your birthing journey will be one of you and your intention and one that pervades challenges. Building a sense of confidence that consumes you when you need it most, and believing that the strength within you to birth a baby. With comfort and ease. As the ability to confidently and calmly navigate, challenges overcome them, with the ability to control and calm your mind, your energy and body into alignment, bringing forth a definite ability to birth your baby with confidence and ease. And feel less pain. Actively turning pain into pleasure.

Birthing babies encourages mothers to birth in their chosen way. They have overcome challenges in their beliefs their environments and made changes in their perceptions so they can more fully accept who they are. To overturn what they previously thought and believed true and embrace a new concept of childbirth, of themselves as a mother, a woman, and a lover.

What you learn here will expand into all areas of your life so you can literally change the course of your life for the better while absorbing what you read. Life can be good. This resonating and resounding through your life, will encourage a path that changes the alignment, brings you confidence and will provide you with solutions, as if by magic.

It brings them through your life as simple stepping stones which you can easily navigate with a sense of calm composure and grace. Including Pregnancy and childbirth.

Your pregnancy journey is unique there are obvious commonalities and likenesses between women, your body is your own, your vision is your own and your birth is your birth, your babies birth is your birth story as yet unwritten. To be defined by you. The birth plan is one thing, but your choice to determine how you feel and experience birth is different, you can control the logistics to some extent, but you can more effectively control the way you determine your experience inside. And that is what is most important "Birthing babies with the big O" is a contemporary, empowering and upbeat, guide to birthing your baby with multiple streams of relief. To include the orgasmic template of union in birth as you will uncover, to birth baby in the most natural way intended. Building confidence, to redefine your relationship with your body and arousal and bringing this into birth, in an elegant and dignified way.

It's a journey in and of itself and will represent a commitment to you. To change something and to be something that makes your life good. Bringing the most up to date personal empowerment evolutions and the leading insights on the biochemistry of birth and how it can be elegantly merged with the orgasmic template to bring pleasure and efficiency to the birthing suite.

Using education, relaxation and visualisation into child birth together with scientific developments in the management of pain using, arousal, to accompany you and guide you through child birth.
It is an educational journey, aimed to build strengths, confidences, so you are qualified capable and strong. To define your child birth path as you choose. Designed and authored by World Class Personal Empowerment Expert Victoria Whitney.

In person she has a strength and calm essence in addition to her wealth of experience the vibrancy and energy she has are unique. The way she works is mysterious, but when you look backward in 6 months time you will notice that you have changed and there is something very different, palpably so and it was almost effortless. This is one of the great strengths to being worked with by Victoria.

Do you have time for the practice in this book? Can you make 20 minutes each day, if it was to enhance the course of your forever, Bring great things in ways that you do not even know yet.

The answer is inevitably yes. so read on.

We all have 24 hour days.

But when you choose to take 10, twenty minutes for purpose it can literally change your life.

The journey you and baby will take together will have highs and lows. There will be moments when you doubt there will be moments of immense joy. The doubts will signal change. All of which will begin to come together as you work through the pages of this book. The journey is augmented by " Birthing

babies - Hypnotherapy for Childbirth. The Ultimate Guide To Positively Empowered Birth.
 ***There are four guided visualisations included in this book. To read these to yourself into a digital recorder or access the pre recorded sessions available (link in Acknowledgements) ***

It's early days but this is the perfect time to envision, and learn. As you read through the next chapters what you learn will become a welcome truth for you, and you will begin to appreciate the shift in resonance is vital now. To define the next steps for your birth and the possibility that you have choice in how you observe your labour, and your birth. How you feel it, how you experience it, and most of all how you can influence it.

How to use this book. Take an open mind and absorb what you choose. What is right for you will naturally permeate your life. The journey of pregnancy will draw on you in ways you can not even imagine but when you are at the point where you need it, you will always have everything you need inside to do the thing that you thought you couldn't do. The big O is another layer of confirmation that you really do have everything you need inside to make life good. To birth your baby confidently and feel less pain.

Life is going to change in some of the most beautiful and challenging ways. The secret is right here, you are now directing that change. That is the difference. It's true that life will never be the same again and that's a good thing. Whether planned and expected, or unplanned and unexpected. You're reading this book because you're choosing your path for birthing baby and motherhood with intention.
You have a whole lifetime ahead of you. And that is an opportunity which should never daunt you. It is totally possible to make sure from the very first thought that it is in alignment with the real vision you have for yourself as a mother or a father and as a women or man. And that is a gentle process of simply being aware. Honestly I believe and know that everyone can be empowered to have the life they envisioned, the opportunities experiences, for themselves and their family, all it takes is deliberation and intention. Anyone can (including

me)
 And that kind of unwavering faith. Many women at this time are dawning a new consciousness of determination of natural birth without intervention or asserting the scope of the mind body connection and the bond between mind and body that has always existed. To use it to recognise it. We're all for intervention when it is necessary but most times we pray and hope that it does not become a requirement. That said we are more for the women to handle the prospect of it in a way that they know they are enough. With it or without. So much of our lives people feel determined by others, by circumstances, by the world, things that are outer to our control. But you realise sometime within, sometime in life, preferably now that the most control you have is here in the now. This is the time. So to continue to pursue the knowledge and education which enables you to to birth your baby the way you want, to choose how you birth, into the life you desire. To birth baby with confidence. Birth baby with love. And birth yourself into a phenomenal mother. This is the time.

You can absorb new ideas, explore different ways different concepts right here right now and each and every one will shift something to support you. As you work through this text, you will be reminded to your strengths. There is new knowledge but mostly this is a reminder. You to bring strength and supportive choices it will building faith in trust between you and you. Your mind and body your mind and soul. Or quite simply to birth your baby as naturally as possible. It will at the most basic level shift some fears, educate you in some details you had previously known which will bring value to you at some time in some place in some space in the future without doubt.

Many women want a natural birth without intervention. For whatever reason, and now you can learn the simple way of the how to do that. It can't be promised because even with all of the planning in all of the world, birth is birth. And can take unforeseen paths, the difference is in how you interpret, experience and respond in these moments .

You have the scope of the mind body connections and the bond between mind and body that has always existed coherently forever. To use this connection harness, it learn it and evolve into and through it, to birth baby calmly and confidently. The Big O is more than the mind body connection, we highlight a new and dynamic shift in the perception of the female body its origination. Its design, perfection and form. Asking the unaskable questions like, why do women have a clitoris, is it purely for pleasure or was it purposed for the role of pain relief aswell.

Merging accepted constructs, pivotal in labour and pregnancy, the three c's Calm, confident and in control. They are the underlay of birthing babies. Here we add a fourth. Climax. When you are calm confident and in control, it seems like the everything. You are present. Nothing else matters. When you are calm, confident and in control you always have control, not of the environment necessarily, but you have control of your mind and your body.
Your thoughts and the way the chemical makeup of your body responds to how you receive the environment.
You have this silent power. It's a palpable strength you have when you remain calm. You have the choices you have the bond you have the beautiful bond with baby. And it supports you in staying calm confident and in control and making sure your intentions and needs through the progression of your life are fulfilled. Bringing the fourth C into the paradigm brings a whole new window of possibility. The introduction of the fourth C to bring a further dimension to the reduction of the pain paradigm. To bring together and synergise the science behind birth and the calm competence mental prowess and focus to build a very strong formula for childbirth with less pain.

For example. Your baby is grown within you, you don't need to tell your body how to do it because it already knows. You maybe require reminder occasionally that you do know what to do, just like your body knows what to do.

You will experience the simple fleeting acceptances within you, every cell of your body aligning with its natural purpose and growing baby, without thought purposefully guiding you to nutrients and actions and internal and external actions and support mechanisms that will nourish baby within you. It's astounding, we don't even think it down to this level. You have it. You are it. You do it. A complete life support unit for a growing human. And it's host.

With that competence. If that doesn't inspire you to believe in yourself I don't know what will. You are growing the cellular connections that will support baby for the whole nine months, and it's entire life, and prepare your body for birthing baby.

In the early pregnancy days it is natural to feel tired, it's a tiredness you will have never known, like bone tired, it's called growth. You are establishing the infrastructure to sustain, so much.

Knowing you were born with the ability to immaculately build this infrastructure is incredible in and of itself. What else are you capable of. What else, latent until you need it. Much like many inherent assets you have.

Exploring the fascinating latencies of your body, and calm you into a confident birth, giving you the ability to manage your level of comfort by uncovering and engaging a new layer of hidden truths about your body. Would you be made with the degree of intricacy that you have been, to the ability to make such exacting calculations that keep your baby alive, without being afforded the ability to manage the pain that accompanies the birth of your child. It's somehow doubtful. To one perspective you can synthesise that in nature most components for drugs are found from, at some stage in their development, raw plant herbal base. Even when this taken as a template and reproduced in a pharmacological form.

The infrastructure of all nature, inspires our progression as man no matter how we distance ourselves from it through pharmacological advances. Even industrial development. You just have to look at the intricacy of nature in detail to see the patterns we take for granted, in industrial development. Ferrous wire, Steel cabling used in everything, buildings, transport a dominant component in our progressive life, reflects in the intricacy of the body of a sand eel as just one small example. It's all hidden in nature. And you are nature.

In this context, we may encroach on the areas unspoken. The areas taboo. But that's clear in the title. The areas that could potentially wield one of the most significant advancements in feminine empowerment in birth.

The very idea of Orgasmic Birth, does sound cosmic but it does not have to be.

There is a reason you are reading this book. It may be because you are curious, You can note your reason, your why, it's important. I can give you all the reasons in the world just roll them off one by one, but they will be meaningless. Because they are not yours, what are your real reasons. You have chosen to research natural birth, you are pregnant and bored so you are reading, and this is baby related so it seemed a good fit. You are a midwife expanding your knowledge. Whatever your reason that will form the basis for your interpretation of this book but also the efficacy of the techniques. When you are invested personally with emotion to realise the reasons you are here, for a more natural birth, reduced medication, to learn new techniques. All of the above. Your reasons are important valid and should be heard by you. Make a note of them. They are a guiding force a beacon for you. When you are personally invested you have faith, hope another layer that supports you. And that makes a difference.

There is a reason you have chosen to find education to influence your birthing path forward. Allot of the principles in this book will spread out in waves through your life like ripples. Birthing baby can be a very powerfully positive experience. It can feel good.
Women aren't sold this image by the media but it is the real truth. Labour does not have to be laboric. By allowing yourself the space to think about what you want, what can go well and also being prepared for the inevitable things don't always go well. Having a solution there already lined up ready to present itself at the right time. "Birthing babies" and 'Birthing babies with the Big O " will give you the feeling of control. The point in principle is when you are pregnant it is a place of vulnerability. But also great strength. There are so many unknowns, so you make a plan, a bigger birth plan, the most common feeling of being led by the system is very very common. You are included in this plan as are your own desires around what you want your birth to be, and how you choose to experience your level of comfort. That your body is your own and your choices, are heard, foremost by you. And all is possible in dignity.

CHAPTER TWO

" Even with the awkwardness of first time love, there was a grace and purity, carnal and beautiful that I knew I could not live without " Fiona Zedde

What is an orgasm.

And illusive isn't an acceptable answer. Excepting they aren't as elusive as you may believe is a good start point. They aren't illusive you can experience them. They are real, they are good and they are within you.

Oxfords English Dictionary

noun: orgasm; plural noun: orgasms

1. the climax of sexual excitement, characterized by intensely pleasurable feelings centred in the genitals and (in men) experienced as an accompaniment to ejaculation.

"she managed to achieve an orgasm"

Some people squirm at the question and the very word. It's not something we talk about openly over coffee in Britain and quite appropriately it's a very private experience. The very word makes people blush, because it is a deeply personal experience. And very context specific and dependent, it's a deeply personal identification, definition, story, and experience. In discussion, people often have to associate into thinking of the experience to be able to reference mentally what you are saying, to make sense of the concept, so say orgasm and the human mind is naturally drawn to think of their own orgasms, at some level. So, it makes people blush. But were talking new ground here, the science, and the sequence of orgasm relative to birth. Everyone is different, yet everyone can experience and use orgasmic birthing practices, and feel calm, confident and in control. To learn to enhance this experience is something more refined, and something beautiful, and acceptance of self and an acceptance of your femininity. The natural temptation is to be imagining scenarios and assumptions of pornographic, routines, deep pleasure, and multiple orgasms in the bedroom. This is a distance from the re conceptions of the birthing suite as a place of arousal. A distance in understanding and education of the space between that place within you and bridging the gap between there and you, and the instinctive application of orgasms in potentially the most valuable and valid context yet. Childbirth. The greatest distinction here is the difference between sex, and intimate acts with a partner, and a woman becoming so in tune with her own sensuality, and primal nature to harness the frequency of arousal independently, to move through birth with less pain and more pleasure. This is a leap, but a leap you can evolve to take. The difference in the frequency or resonance between the two grades of intimacy and arousal, is great. The beautiful thing is that you can maintain both. Alongside the great depth of your intimate relationship with your partner, or partners. You are building space for you as a woman to foster a new facet within yourself to allow for that transition. Where you can expand your own sexuality to encompass and include labouring with self-love and arousal. By learning the value, the reason and then yourself piecing these together to merge your own sense of what is acceptable. All enshrined within the context and intention of birthing baby with greater ease, comfort, and pleasure.

So many layers of preconception or association will be overcome for you to have a new attachment to the internal meaning or identification you give to orgasmic pleasure.

Working from the basics.

The sequence of arousal and climax.

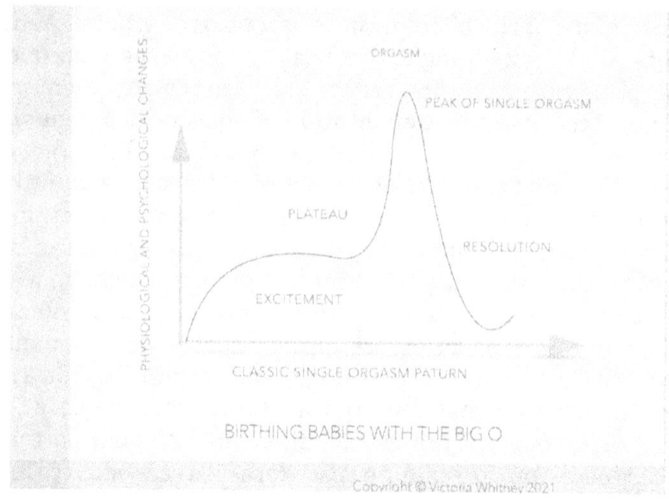

Beginning ...

The Excitement.

The thing is you don't even need to touch someone. This can be a look, a touch, a stroke, a tender kiss, the beginnings of arousal build through each sensual layer, touch taste sense, smell, all building, signalling the rise in the heart rate, respiration, and blood pressure. Muscle tension, skin becomes flushed nipples become hardened. Flushed and invigorated blood flow increases to the genitals, swelling of the female labia minora, and vaginal lubrication. Breasts begin to swell.

With mental focus it is possible to engage these sensations without even touching anyone or even yourself, just mentally induct them. By visualising and imagining. In order to do so you may choose to make a quiet new corner of your mind to do so. Where no one else can go.

The sense of anticipation is enough to build the sensations of arousal. The beginnings. To imagine can invoke the biochemical hormonal lead trail that precedes orgasm.

Plateau.
The changes in phase 1 begin to intensify. The vagina continues to swell the increased blood flow and vaginal walls turn dark purple. The woman's clitoris becomes highly sensitive

and retracts under the clitoral wall to avoid direct stimulation.
As the stimulation of the erogenous zones continues and increases.
Muscle tension increases.

Orgasm.
Involuntary muscle spasms increase, blood moves to the extremities and engorges pleasure centres which excites the nerve endings increasing the sense of arousal. A series of rhythmic contractions occur in the uterus vagina and pelvic floor muscles the feeling of warmth spreads through the entire body especially the pelvis area. With mental excitement and invigoration.

Resolution.
The body relaxes and blood flows away from the engorged areas. Women can begin again within minutes and re-engage with stimulation and repeat the cycle.

Enhanced by a general sense of wellbeing and enhanced intimacy, often fatigue. Some (most - all) women are capable of a rapid return to further stimulation and may frequently experience multiple orgasms in sequence.

The more you practice this cycle, the more you can maintain the pleasure platform for longer periods of time and increase the effectiveness and efficacy of stimulation. Especially when the purpose and attachment is to prolong the pleasure sensations, learning and embedding the mental and physical sense and flooding your nervous systems pain receptors with the alternate and opposite chemical, hormonal load. To do this mental control is also required but we will approach this in a later chapter.

The attachment and association are to support you in achieving and prolonging pleasure, and climax so you can birth baby more comfortably.

There are many ways you can achieve orgasm.

Each has its own strength, which will be brought together when we assimilate and synergise the mutual efficiency of arousal, climax, the female anatomy, and the sequence of labour. Centrally, climax and pleasure so you can birth baby more comfortably.

Clitoral

To pace your own experience of pain. By massaging the clitoris gently in a way that you are familiar with to increase pleasure, as you internally fixate on comfort in labouring and pleasure the dichotomy suggests that the pain will be overtaken by pleasure. Imagining a wave of pleasure however you choose, such as a colour or the realisation of the Imagination of your body releasing overriding chemicals that bring ease comfort and flow.

Euphoria exists within the body so imagining of the body birthing baby is the intention to lace around your climactic visualisations when in labouring form. What defines your experience is your motive.

Primarily the an important definition is to distinguish between sexual acts with a lover adn their motive and sexual acts for the purposes of birthing baby. The motive is different, and your attention directive is different here you are intending for the expansion of pleasure sensations within your body with the intention of birthing baby as the time to labour comes. So, the sense of longing desire, is different, because it is a sense that the desire is within for the sensation of pleasure and acknowledging your ability to manifest the pleasure independently in your mind as well as your body. This is met with the realisation of comfort, and core independence. So learning to centre your mind and thoughts on your body and the sensations of pleasure within, is a something that you can engage in and learn to do. You are the centre of your mind, your body and your thoughts and actions and your attention is centred on pleasure in the context of learning to increase the sensation of pleasure in birth. Your body is once again your friend. It's structure and perfect form whatever shape and size you are or worship.

The structure of the clitoris is evaluated in the next chapter. But as a forerunner, It has over 10,000 receptors, nerve endings. No study has yet quantified the number of nerve fibers (axons) that suffuse (invigorate) the human clitoris. The dorsal nerves of the clitoris (DNCs) are the primary source of sensation and somatic clitoral inclusion. The dorsal nerve runs forward first in the pudendal canal above the internal pudendal (nerve that supplies sensation) vessels and then in the deep perineal space between these vessels and the pubic arch. The clitoris is in truth 11 centimeters long and has its own erectile tissues. Mostly hidden in the vaginal walls and beneath the perinium. As such you can imagine the sensations of the sensations of arousal forming a path forming a wave.

The use of clitoral stimulation is adjusted to 'match' the intensity of contractions, so that pleasure overrides the discomfort, their strength is great though so are the intuitive senses that lead you to match the intensity. The more you are aware of your body you are aware of the sense of comfort and pleasure measuring the sense of progress instinctively knowing where to pace and where to lead. The difference between pleasuring in an intimate context, when having sex and in foreplay is different. Here you are intentionally bringing arousal for the purposes of birthing baby and harmonising the environment of your body in one main intention to feel less pain. The instinct and rawness will feel different. The intention. To override the pain sensors with pleasure and synergise the labouring process with orgasm. This concept alludes to the previously discussed theory that the brain cannot respond to pain and pleasure simultaneously, and that when one sensation is predominant, the other is reduced (Arms, 1994)

Vaginal – vaginal orgasms are rare and less easy to achieve in context, though definitely possible. This takes deep penetration, with resulting deeper orgasm, deeper meaning cervical, where the entire musculature seated within the clitoris stretches beneath the surface of the vaginal opening and behind, the depth of orgasm is compounded by the inclusion of the stimulation and awakening of the clitoral crura, becomes a very deep and very intense orgasm. This includes excitement of the front vaginal wall, which is home to the anterior fornix or "a" spot. When pressure is focused on the front wall of the vagina there is a marked increase in pleasure sensations.

Though every woman is different - Deep penetration is not advised during labour. This said Cervical orgasms have the intensity of the pleasure lasting longer than other orgasms. Since the cervix is at the lower end of your uterus and what sets labour forward is the pressure forming from uterine contractions once this process starts the cervix is engaged in childbirth and no longer a role in orgasm by stimulation but to feel the sensations of relaxation and mounting pleasure from the clitoris and surrounding vaginal structures and sensory points. The climactic waves can bring harmony to the cervix, but then you imagine its role in childbirth it is to expand, effacement is the thinning of the cervix and expansion, there has been a plug a mucus plug formed and traversing the opening to the uterus, a barrier between baby and the vaginal opening so that it remains free of infection once the plug begins to efface and leave the body the vaginal cavity is to be approached with the attitude and approach of sterility and gentility.

On the whole cervical orgasms are much more holistic much deeper and more intense. They stimulate the cervix, vaginal walls, and the clitoral structures both inside hidden beneath the vaginal opening the perinium and directly behind the opening of the vagina. When this network is enlivened, you can imagine the sensations of potential when you begin to visualise the network in harmony all merging together in synergistic form like each part of a wave of ignition of desire and pleasure, like dominos, or a mexican wave on wave of pulsation of biochemical inductions paced with intention to expand the pleasure sensations, causing the uterine structures to pulsate and contract in climactic waves. Within the harmonic web of arousal. When you arouse the clitoris and vaginal walls this will affect a deep sense of pleasure wave through the cervical structures and bring more comfort and malleability to these structures. When you are relaxed at home and have a sense of safety, trust. They are more flexible, the can stretch and expand more easily The sensation of familiarity when you are labouring in a space of safety and comfort, makes using all these prospective forms of pleasure an advantage. This is building a plane of existence for you as a woman to foster a new facet within yourself to allow for that transition. Where you can expand your own sexuality to encompass and include labouring with self-love and arousal. By learning the value, the reason and then yourself piecing these together to merge your own sense of what is acceptable. All enshrined within the context and intention of birthing baby with greater ease, comfort, and pleasure.

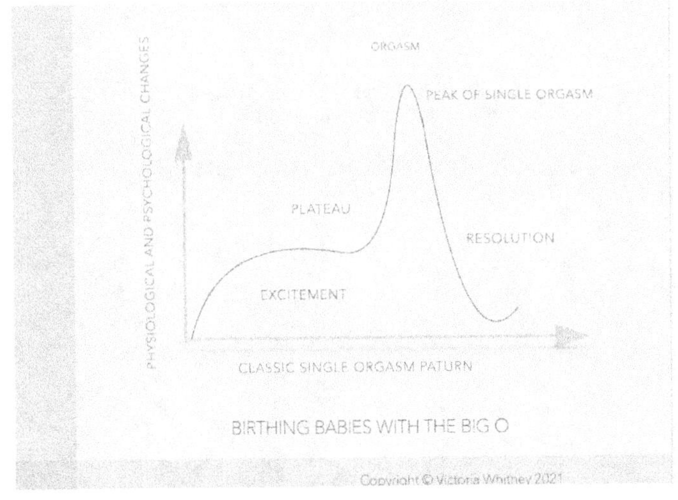

CHAPTER THREE

Welcome to Your vagina
It is beautiful

A gateway to life

We are very familiar with the word uterus and cervix, vagina, and clitoris haven't been included in childbirth familiarisation since the intimate act where baby was made. However, the science behind your clitoris and the influence of waves of pleasure on the sensation of pain is astounding. The facts do not need to be sold to you because with your own mind you can induce the possibilities. So, as you work through these pages I lay down the facts.

The Clitoris

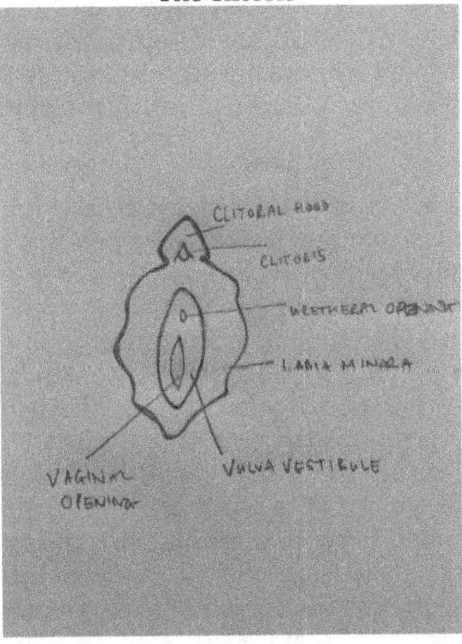

The clitoris is only beginning to be understood to be appreciated and to be accepted as a central pleasure point. It also has the unique distinction of being the only organ in the human body dedicated solely to pleasure, an amazing fact that has ironically been left neglected by science for many years. Not only has the clitoris been largely ignored throughout history, information about it — when given — has often been partial or plainly incorrect.

In the 1400s, a guide considered the clitoris the "devil's teat," and any woman with one was a witch. That females were denied the concept of. Pleasure and that it was to be largely ignored and hindered even removed. Female pleasure was taboo. Where the pleasure of a woman was denied because in gave her strength and carnal desire in the perception of the clergy and all righteous men. Even in the early 20th century, Freud was convinced a woman's ability to orgasm was based on her psychological maturity and that only mentally healthy women could have vaginal orgasms. He did however make an awful lot of fame and fortune in his determination to hystericalise women, in their time, when quite possibly what would have grounded them and brought about sanity was to engage with and accept their sexual nature and embrace their bodies as their own. In a time when women became hysterical was because they were thought as a commodity of man for the purpose of pleasuring man like embellished dolls. Chattels. When in fact they were awakened women with education and entertainment of their intelligence but not passions. They in-turn became hysterical. They had no way to channel their creative passions.

Ignorance about the clitoris is dwindling but it is still something so hidden so taboo. It's your own personal place for exploration and enjoyment your personal pleasure centre alongside all the other centres in life. Becoming confident enough to appreciate enjoy and talk about the clitoris - and how it functions is a birth right for you as a woman, and learning how to enhance your own sexual pleasure through knowledge is your birth right and the path of true education. The good news is that the tide is shifting. It's shifting so women are confident to seek education to learn to explore their bodies and the more women know even teenage girls the more they are aware and the greater safety and confidence they will have. To embrace education and to do so from a standpoint of respecting their bodies themselves before they look to others too early to experiment and regret in the ignorance of their own self-worth and ability to claim their body as their own in a dignified and empowered way. To accept exploration and enjoyment is natural and in fact is more beneficial is a confidence a young woman should have to enjoy her body before she shares it. The Clitoris is not the only centre though a centre that has between 8000 and 10, 00 nerve endings, erectile tissue muscle and nerve endings – whereas the vaginal walls have little sensation at all in comparison. It is also the only part of the human body that never ages, it has one single purpose and that is pleasure. We have our own predesigned pain-relieving centre right there and it has been ignored and forbidden for centuries and in many cultures still is. Where is it sits above the ureteral opening and behind the clitoral hood. It measures 1 centimetre long, most of which is inside the body. And presents like a pea shaped form on the exterior The vulva vestibule signals the gateway to the vagina all sur-rounded in nerve endings which manifest pleasure.

Before moving to the vagina. The vagina The lower part of the vaginal opening called the " A spot " The anterior fornix. This is the most sensitive part of the vagina. And of course the famous G spot (less practically accessible in birthing. But potentially very helpful if baby leaves the birth canal at the exact correct angle.) Other erogenous zones,

The lips

The neck

The ear lobes

Inner thighs

Inner wrist

Nipples

Mouth

The area behind the knees

The perineum

The upper and lower back

Hands

Belly button.

All these places can be stimulated to increase the production of oxytocin and the endorphins the cause the sensations of orgasm and reduce sensations of pain. Is by self-stimulation or gentle manipulation by you, a partner for even using sexual enhancement aids. All the above can apply. Ideally it is within your own control. You are learning to merge and balance the sensations of pain and pleasure within. Which is likely something that you would choose to do alone.

Touch is not even required for arousal. Simply the building anticipation, brings the sensation of arousal to the body and can be harnessed by a visualisation and reigned for the intention of birthing baby. As a woman who has command of her own desires and her sexuality and sensuality to birth baby with greater ease.

It's important to define the distinction between sex for pleasure and eroticism the bedroom, the rawness and decadence of intimacy purely for pleasure, and arousal intending orgasms in birth, the intention is very different, and it's graced with a very different tone. This is building a platform for you as a woman to foster a new facet within yourself to allow for that transition. Where you can expand your own sexuality to encompass and include labouring with self-love and arousal. By learning the value, the reason and then yourself piecing these together to merge your own sense of what is acceptable. All enshrined within the context of complete acceptance and intention of birthing baby with greater ease, comfort, and pleasure.

Wrapped around it is a sentiment of bringing the very deepest of intimacy and vulnerability, to the forefront of a woman's birthing experience.

It is a time when all women feel vulnerable, no matter how strong and confident. There is a challenge to balance the vulnerability with great strength, to accept that the unfamiliar untrodden path may be the one that leads to the absolute realisation of a birth with no pain. A birth with less pain, into a possession of the woman within herself to encompass a new acceptance for this distinction. To accept herself.
To bring about pleasure such that she can birth her baby with greater ease and confidence.

The vagina is just one part of the female sexual system – the muscular opening in the female pelvis, from the external genitals (the vulva) to the cervix, the opening to the internal female reproductive system. The vagina is an important part of the female sexual system, allowing pleasurable forms of penetration. Internal stimulation is a pleasurable part of many women's sexual experience. Many women, however, do not experience orgasm through penetration alone. For maximum pleasure, all of the above can apply.

The entrance to the vagina, called the entroitus, is a hive of pleasure centres.
The vagina itself isn't very sensitive, but of course internal stimulation can be highly pleasurable. You can reach the roots of the clitoris that extend back into the body. On the top wall of the vagina, towards the clitoris, you can find the female prostate, sometimes called the g-spot or skene's gland.
It's possible for baby to directly align with the g spot and meet it on its way through the birth canal as occurs in spontaneous orgasms.

Once you turn your perspective, you and see the whole birth as a very sensual experience. And you can make it more so by accepting your ability to sensualise it. Some women experience spontaneous orgasms on delivery. When the baby's head touches the G spot as it passes through the birth canal. By this time it is too late to experience the full benefits of the orgasmic pleasure which sits in the window between the initiation of contractions and birth itself. That's the full capacity of what you can achieve. Most complications can arise or be amplified by stressors. When you cannot promise of a zero intervention birth you can prepare and do everything you can, everything possible to minimise the risk of intervention. And The Big O is just one of those things.

By reflecting the clitoris, for one single organ to be present with one purpose. It is curious that such an organ does exist and that it has not been assigned in our evolved world a purpose other than sexual or intimate pleasure. Long cast and even judged, mutilated, because its purpose was pleasure. How different the perception that a hub of pain-relieving sensation. A completely new purpose for an anatomical individuation. Perfectly aligned conceptually with childbirth.

Though the female body does have many centres for arousal that are not intimate areas, they are intimately touched, caressed, though are not perceived as imitate. But party to an intention of arousal.

The role of the cervix in orgasms is limited though the cervix is centralised as a gateway to the uterus with protective essences to ensure the uterus is protected in pregnancy.

During the months of pregnancy, the cervix protects your baby with a mucus plug forming barrier that protects the uterus from infection. As labour draws close the mucus plug begins to dissolve sparked by the sensation of the pressure on the inner side of the cervix by the engagement of baby.

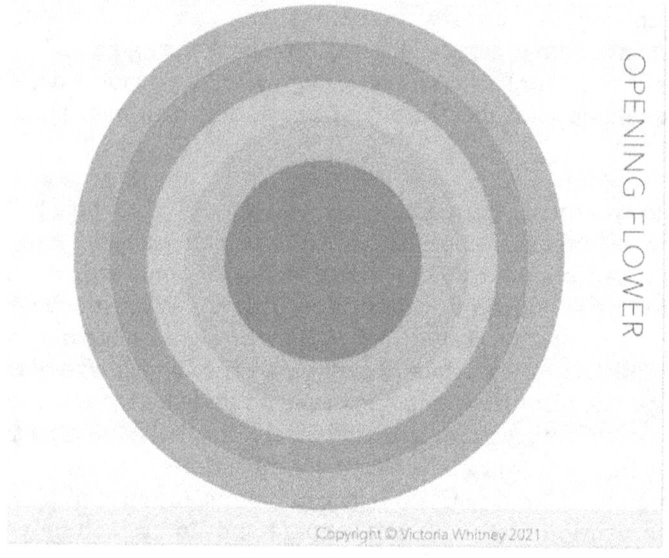

Just as importantly - Your uterus.
Its an Entire world.

It's functional purpose as well as a sexual organ. It's role in child birth is phenomenal. If you idealise what is actually possible and reflect what your body is capable of it makes the concept of arousal bringing pain relief as if it was your natural design, more acceptable and actually you can't not begin to see that it is the right thing to do.

The uterus. It is so intelligent. The human reproductive system is so immaculately ordained. How can we not believe it doesn't have everything we need to birth baby with comfort. As far as organs go our hearts beat and our lungs breathe but actually your uterus grows small human along with the support and cohesion of our other organs. It grows an actual person. Immaculately and that's what it is programmed to do to create a life support system for baby. With that known idea that childbirth without fear is pre programmed into your body to just do it. As long as we stay out of the way. Breathe, relax, and work with our body it can do it.

Just the dimensions and facts... 14 inch muscular purse ½ inch think. At 16 weeks gestation it sits 2 inches below navel. At 23 weeks its peak is at navel. At 7 months 2- 3 inches above the navel. At 38 weeks highest point in abdomen and then at 40 weeks drops 2 inches as head engages and water reduces.

Foetal development.

At 12 weeks: most organs are formed. 14 weeks: doctors can tell the sex of the foetus. 16 to 20 weeks: you may be able to feel movement. 24 weeks: the foetus has a chance of survival outside the uterus.

Perhaps the most self less act of the unthinking uterus without ego it makes sure that baby develops as quickly and safely as possible so that it can thrive without it. In just over half its predicted use time. Just 24 weeks in the event of emergency there it is. It has skills and it works them. Throughout that whole time. Living. breathing. Circulating. Giving life and taking waste a way. Every moment of every day.

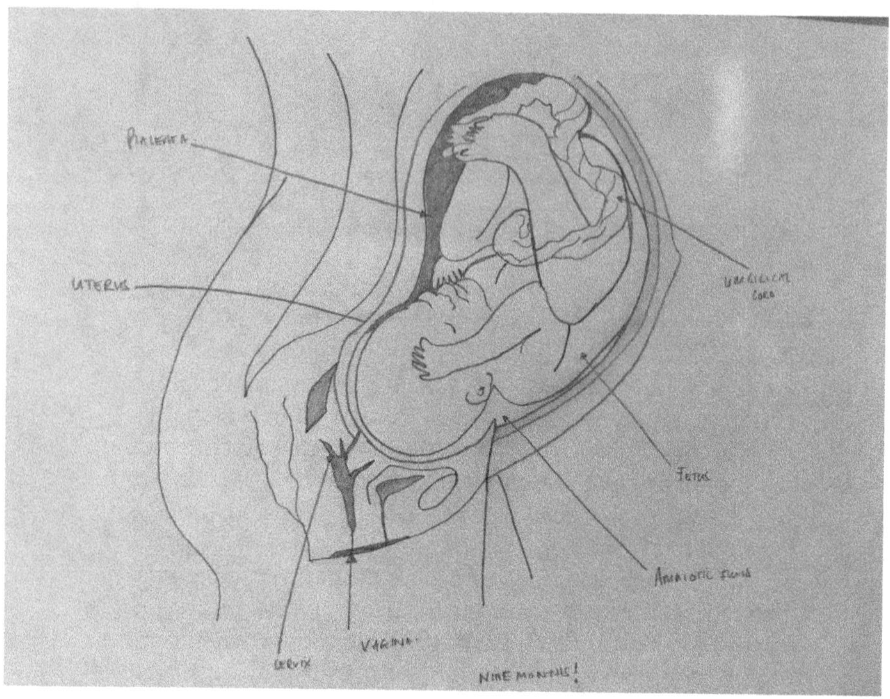

Our uterus grows a small human from and egg and a sperm and sustains it through 9 months of growth and development into a small person. Perfectly formed.
Just a womb. Just a place of safety for your growing foetus but it is so much more. The value in knowing this is great. Because its an example of just one thing that goes on behind the scenes of our ignorance that is so perfectly innately ordained within us.

Such a beautiful example of the structure that can be weaved by our body and mind in harmony when in reality it's so much more. The structure and the interwoven network that makes that happen is astounding. Each fibre each and every blood vessel uniquely defined and designed to not just withstand but also withhold the growth of a foetus through 9 months. The growth of each and every skin cell every organ and every single cell of baby that forms into its perfectly organized human self. The unique infrastructure beautifully supports sustains and grows life. And it's is within you.

Every single cell of their body and every aspect of the self is designed to make this life and when they are signed with the essence of themselves and the miracle of the simplicity that makes their body makes their heart beat. As your body changed it's structure to accommodate the growing foetus so do our minds our bodies our sounds and our future hopes, and what is possible for you too.

You think purer in pregnancy, you put what is best for you into your body by reducing alcohol and anything that is not recommended. You are really in the best shape of your life chemically, while you are pregnant so in the same token you will be believing cleaner, and your body will function better as a vehicle for making what you believe into life.
When you support your body and mind in making the environment in your body that is harmonious with your and babies best health your life will turn to support you.
The uterus provides support with both latitudinal and longitudinal muscles. Weaved like the geographic coordinate system. A mirror of the globe, the world. They weave together to it's Inner layer of figure of 8 mesh fibres which all contract in harmony through contraction in labour and hold stable while baby is growing through the three trimesters. That's 10 whole months. It provides blood and takes away waste product alongside the placenta from it's own exertion in growth on a constant level until the babies birth. It's a cycle of growth and a life in and of itself. With it's own purpose which is very profound and very beautiful. It's a work of art. The Inner layer circular fibres and the longitudinal and latitudinal lines which encase the magnitude of the earth. The womb is exactly the same with muscle fibers both longitudinal and latitudinal which work in cohesion through mexican wave motions your baby through the birth canal. Wave like motions that are mirrored in orgasm.

The infrastructure of the uterus

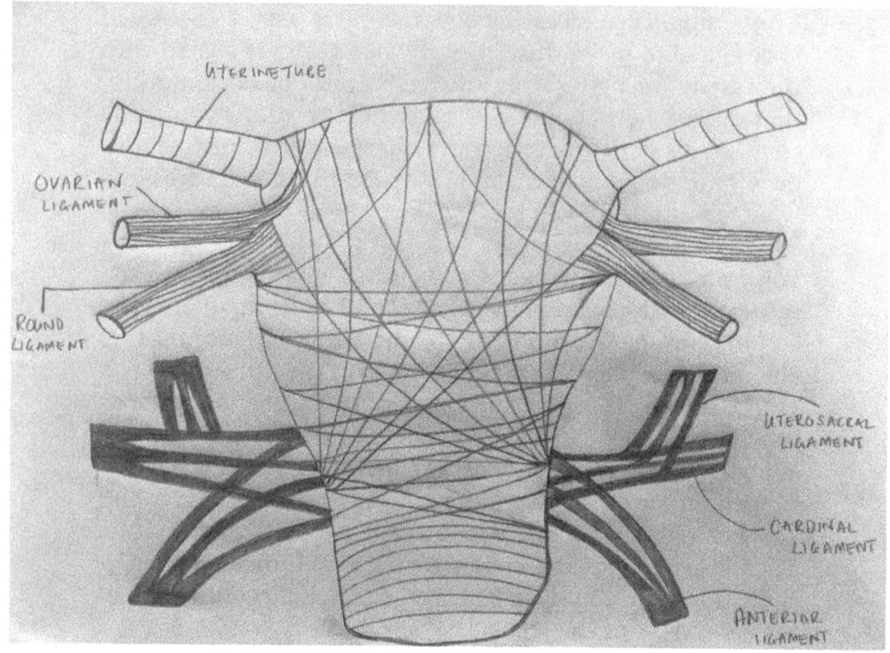

They come in all shapes and sizes each one unique in its form and each one perfect in and of itself. Typically it presents as an upside down pear shape They can be heart shape or variations in between.

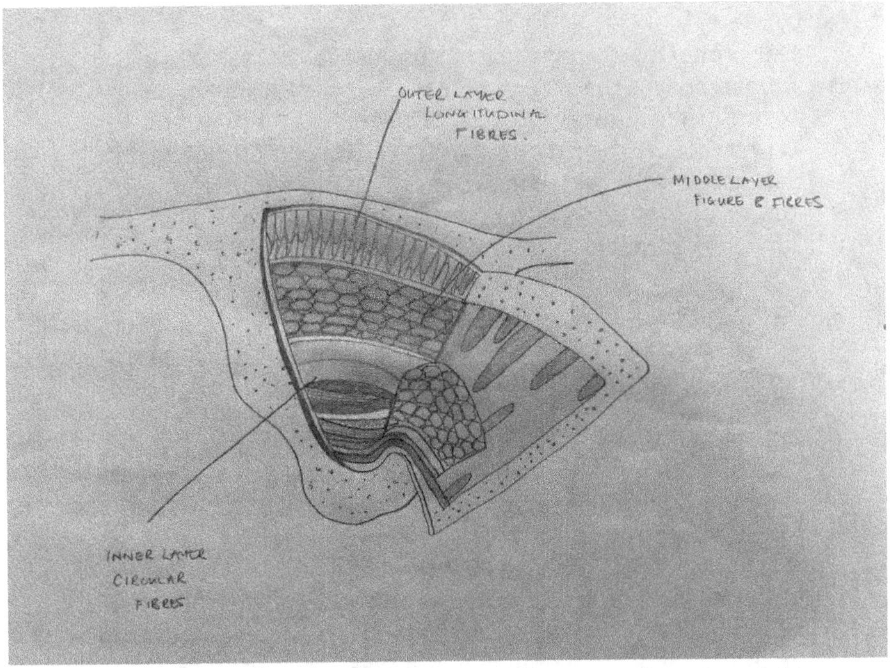

They grow they weave they encircle they encapsulate baby in a space of you and that is so. Spherical and ellipsoidal. They move in a Mexican wave to enable baby to birth through the birth canal ... rhythmic muscle stimulations and sensations as waves of electrical nerve impulses cause a traction. Literally like a wave of movement moving through your body. Something so daunting and so intense can become to appear very simple. The grace and respect of your bodies ability to do that means the main role of your consciousness is to move with the relaxation of your body will allow it to do what its naturally designed to do. The only temptation is to worry and to fear. This is the least effective and last thing you should do. The body is weaved by a artist who demanded perfection at it's creation an artist. Who intricately weaved a web of fine musculature to cradle baby through its term, then wave by wave breath by breath by to electrical nerve impulse to impulse causing the body to contract manifests the birth journey. It's a work of art in its form as your body and a it is a thing of beauty. A thing so great and so magnificent that to simplify it, by the word womb is futile, its immaculate infrastructure is so defined, it's brilliance as it cradles small life, nourishes and in its later stages of term births it into life.

One of the least known but the absolute coolest reflexes in the human body is the Fergusson Reflex. Babies desire to breathe is one trigger in the process of birth. The pressure on the cervix, begins the production of Oxytocin. It stimulates the Fergusson reflex which in turn begins contractions and starts the process of birth. A self sustaining sequence and cycle of uterine contractions - neuro endocrine reflex.

Impressive.

This being true, there can be more purpose for the structure of our sexual organs, in the role of childbirth.
As you lean more about the clitoris you will realise its purpose is greater than it has been previously believed.

Reflecting back to the uterus. When child birth is a reflex.
Your body can do it without your consciousness. So what are you going to choose to do with your consciousness other than support you body in doing what it was created and designed to do by trusting it and loving it and believing in it. There are cases where people in Comas have successfully birthed babies as mentioned below, much as it is sad. The value of these incidences are that your body births baby independently. It knows what to do.

Learning to work with your body staying calm confident and in control, and layer in arousal and climax flush pleasure to out pain. To get our minds out of the way into distraction so that our bodies can do what they need to do to birth baby comfortably and easily.

So if your consciousness turns from fearing and being intimidated by birth to supportive and faithful then how much easier on a whole do you imagine birth can be. It's so simple yet so profound.
And very potent transition. And for the real thinkers its logical to it makes sense. Its not just an airy fairy notion.

Aside, there are examples mostly in the US where women in coma have birthed babies naturally - though they are often with some uncomfortable truth behind them where a woman has been in a coma for several years and yet they have been found to be pregnant and then spontaneously birthed healthy babies. The principle and the case in point is that the body can do this.

Beyond attention to the moral concern that would have caused a pregnancy. Using the guided relaxations, and chapter by chapter layers your mind will be induced to calm and centre scattered thoughts, the doubts and the unknowns to subside, they will calm. Because education brings knowledge and knowledge brings confidence. By alleviating the fears you are redirecting your energy through your body to work with you. Because you will unconsciously without effort experience the building of a force field. Like the uterus for baby but for you and your belief structure, the only difference you can retain this one after birth and it will just get stronger. But it can fully support you. Fully sustain you as you feed it you nourish it. You can fully focus and concentrate on being pregnant and birthing baby.
Birthing baby. Is what your body is designed to do even without thought.
So the only things that sits between you and birthing baby with ease are fears, tensions and the fixation of your attention.

The methods in birthing babies elevate the worries fears and give you ways to channel your attention to assist you in progressing the discomfort and the energy of labour in a way that is beneficial. It is working with your body. Knowing how your body works and also knowing how your energy and attention can all form together to support that is new and great. That being true the only essence that makes labour less easy other than a physical anomaly is fear and tension. According to Hopkins Medical Research Unit at John Hopkins Hospital Only 8% of pregnancies have physical complications. [2] The unknown truth is that Child Birth is a reflex. As you draw closer to your due date, I explain more for this later. The intensity of the oxytocin receptors in your womb increase by 200 fold. This means that your uterus is perfectly primed to react to this hormone. Imagine this was caffeine - and the receptors increased in equal measure. Just imagine. A 200 fold magnification of your morning coffee. This is something I would not want to see, but if you can appreciate the relative difference and the supportive influence of the immaculate design of your body and the birthing process. Then you have a lot of natural anaesthesia already circulating your nervous system encouraging a sense of relaxation and euphoria. Most people don't know this.

You increased the receptors for maximum uptake and maximum effectiveness of the purpose of the hormones. That's a 200 percent magnification to alleviate the tension, relax and expand the muscle fibres and numb the sensation of the expansion, as your baby moves through the birth canal the relaxation and expansion of the fibres all enhanced by the chemical of oxytocin enriching every cell fibre to ease the sensations of expansion and discomfort.

When you imagine the increase in the release oxytocin and the increase in dopamine the flood that comes from natural orgasm is targeted at standard reception in your body when you have a 200 time magnification of the pleasure sensors. Sit with that for a while. Your body is a symphony, there is an internal an orchestra all the instruments playing in symphony and that symphony is you. That's what stimulated the production of oxytocin the contraction of muscles through relaxation of certain muscle groups. Ironically it's the relaxation induced by the love dug oxytocin that brings about the contraction of the muscles. Oxytocin is the love hormone which increases and peaks during arousal.
That progresses the interaction between the uterine wall and the contractions. Its desensitises the parameter walls so that you can reduce the discomfort to allow for the expansion. That progresses the contraction and relaxation of the uterine wall in a Mexican wave to bring about the progression of the baby through the birth canal. Amazing.
Looking back to the Fergusson reflex and your body. The physical process to birth of baby as a reflex. Your body can do this, it has a reflex to initiate contraction and birth baby through the birth canal. This means the one most powerful influence you have is to centralise your mind centralise your thoughts and bring about the fixation of attention. On you being calm confident and in control of your mind, inciting pleasure and comfort and a sense of calm and presence even in the most intense moments, then this is mirrored in your body so that your body can birth baby as was intended by design.

To move with the natural laboric flow. As in natural rhythm with your body.

The word laboric doesn't exist in the English dictionary but as a process or a name to describe a sequence or the entity of a process.

The word as a name laboric even means "You appear strong and powerful. You have an impressive personality and can influence and even intimidate through sheer force" The sheer force of natural birth.

It's a much more effective turn on the phrase labour which has an embrandment of arduous process into a natural flowing sequence. I speak this way though I have experienced full labour. It does require effort and focus and concentration and relaxation and birthing a baby is not quite as effort less as a sneeze. But it is easier when you know what is happening, it is easier when you move with your body, and it is easier when you are aware your body is moving you. And it is much easier when you are calm, confident and in control and climaxing.

In learning a sport it is different, you have to step by step learn an entire new proprioceptive formula of sequential movements.
With child birth it is all seeded unconsciously.
Your body knows what to do.
At this point the presupposition that labour should be arduous is not helpful.
And the chemical makeup in your body counters this suggestion. It is our resistance and preconception that it has to be hard work that makes the process heavy and laboric. But it really isn't so.

The uterus is where life begins, so naturally were working with it, " The big O ' isn't just about making orgasms its about bringing the body to orgasm while it is fulfilling a purpose. The purpose of birthing baby without pain. Counter balancing the pleasure pain sensors into a synonymous rhythm. To birth baby without pain, and to reduce the stress on your physical body.

You see who thought this could make so much sense, orgasms are possible, and you can use them, especially when you time it right. The knowing how to time it will come with faith and exploration. Knowing your body and having faith in your body, your femininity and your confidence and acceptance of self pleasure when in labour. When you can wrap your mind around that as you move through this book then you will be 90% there.

Go ahead with the practical exploration, finding them, having them, and using all of the ways to make sure they are the best ones. (call it Homework !)

So now you know, and can identify What an orgasm is, The stages of orgasm, The layers and how they can translate into the stages of child birth and it actually makes sense when it is overlayed. Call it The orgasmic Template.

The types of orgasm, an introduction to your body, and the places you can make excite to make that happen and how to make them happen. Your uterus - It's intricate structure and the emerging purpose for the orgasmic template.
The stages of labour and what it means to overlay the orgasmic template, through your birthing experience and how to actually do this.

So now you know what an orgasmic birth is, that they are possible, not just spontaneously but when you actually believe that they are possible, and that you can choose to. That you can use your body's own cycles to and chemical trail to overcome discomfort in labour. You are beginning to wrap your head around the possibility that it is an actual real life possibility more so than a joke, or a laughable notion. The sequence of orgasm and arousal, your homework to experiment different scenarios, mentally physically. Different ideas on how to climax experiments. The chemical sequences. How to orchestrate the synergy of your dynamic organic structures and sequences, and how it makes sense so you can use it. You are familiar with your uterus, its role function and form and your erogenous zones, places to try places to learn and places to love.

How can you make this work when you are labouring.

The four stages of labour outlined.
Here is what 9 months gestation looks like within the womb

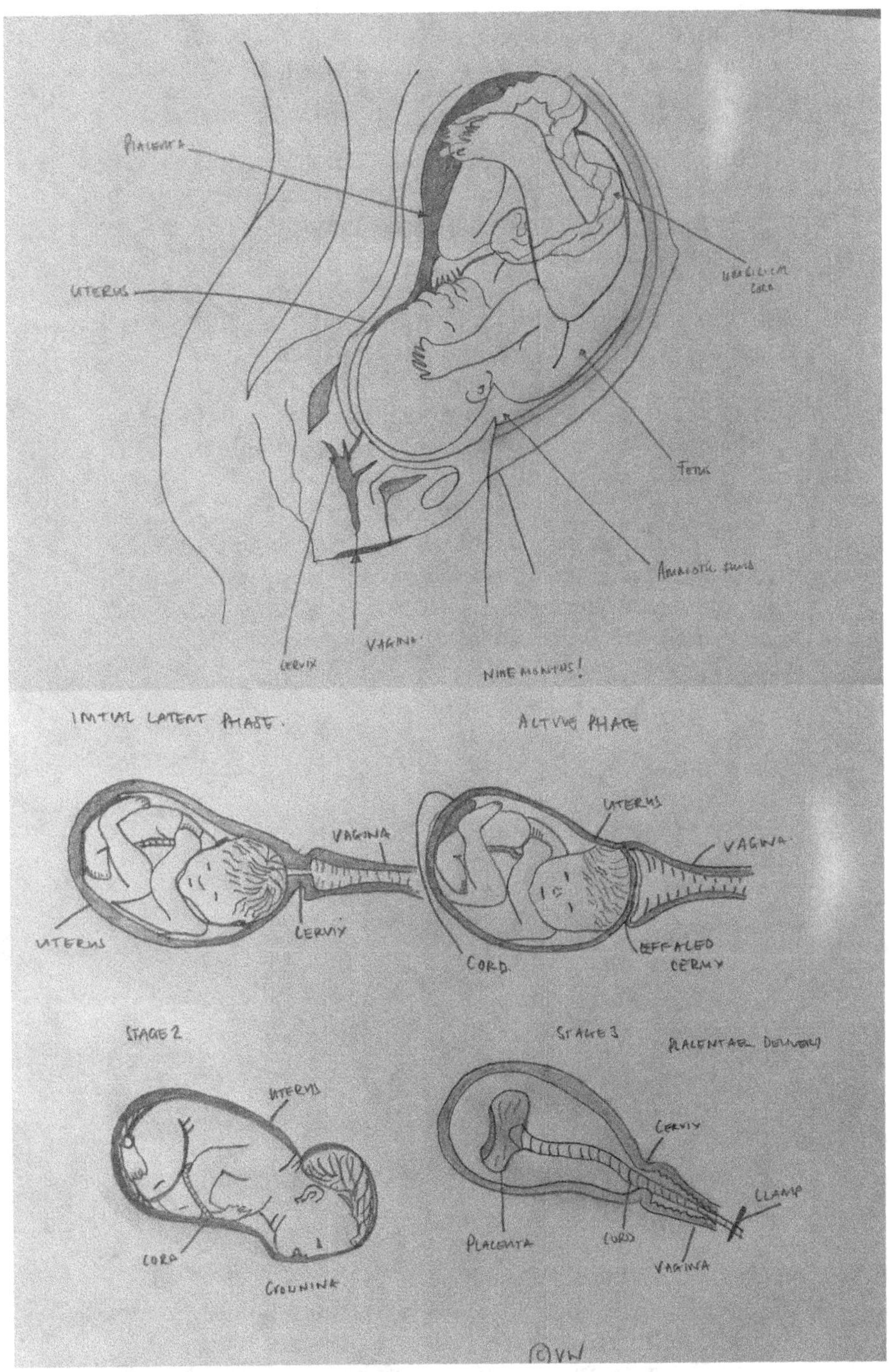

It is cosy but it's beautiful and it's the most connected you will be to anything in your life. Bringing that to the synergy of self-pleasure is a very powerful and humbling connection.

Birth

Beginning with the Latent phase. Low discomfort. The muscles uterine are beginning to relax and wake up, the mucus plug may be dissolved at the cervical cavity and the cervix begins to dilate.

Active phase the lengthening and the dilation of the cervix and movement of baby through the birth canal.

Stage 2 active labour where the pushing begins. All the phases will have their own time frame, and that's individual to you.

Primary stages

The Initial latent stages, the discomfort imagine to be like strong period pain. Feel the sense of comfort by imagining the opening of your cervix by visualising the rings below, each layer represents layers of dilation.

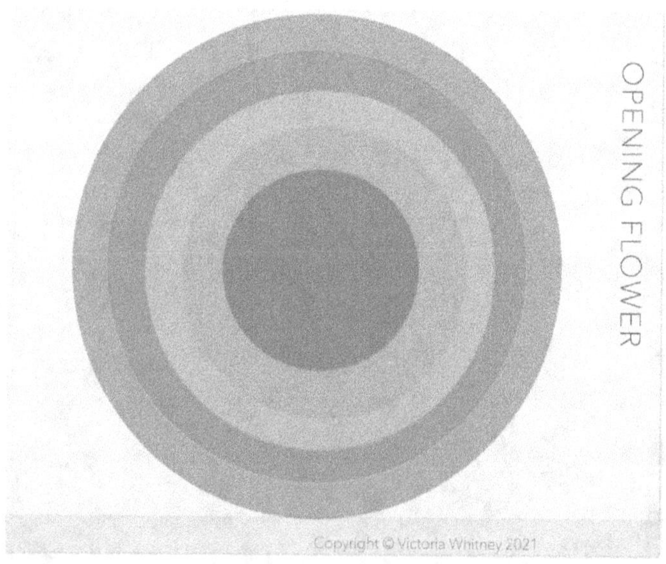

As the cervix lengthens and widens it can be envisioned like the opening of a flower. There is less attention on the cervix currently as its role is different. The importance is your ability to visualise it as an opening, expanding. Comfortably. With the orgasmic template overlayed you will experience and engorgement and a sense of relief and warmth, as the expansion becomes the presence of a feeling of warmth and pleasure, aswell as the sensation of stretching and expansion.

Following engagement, the cervix begins to open following pressure from the uterine contraction. The stages of effacement or thinning of the cervix occur as the uterine contractions, grow stronger.

When you think of contractions and fee fear or trepidation read the paragraph below.

Remembering that contractions at their most intense will be one or just over minutes long and there will be a three minute respite in between. That is sixty seconds of intensity, 180 recovery. When you are labouring those three minutes will feel like a lifetime. That is one minute intense and 3 minutes off. The numbers are in your favour. 3 : 1 rest work ratio. Really that is a favourable ratio when you think about it.

The births you have seen or experienced do not have to form your experience. You can birth differently you can birth in control and you can birth with the orgasmic template.

Remember, when you watch TV the only show the dramatic parts because it is TV.

If the woman arrived in labour sat in a birthing pool very controlled, very quietly to the sound of twinkly music breathed out her baby, the only sound was the harmonious conversation with her birth partner and the first cries of the baby, then got out of the pool dressed and went home. This isn't dramatic enough for TV which is why its so perfect for your life.

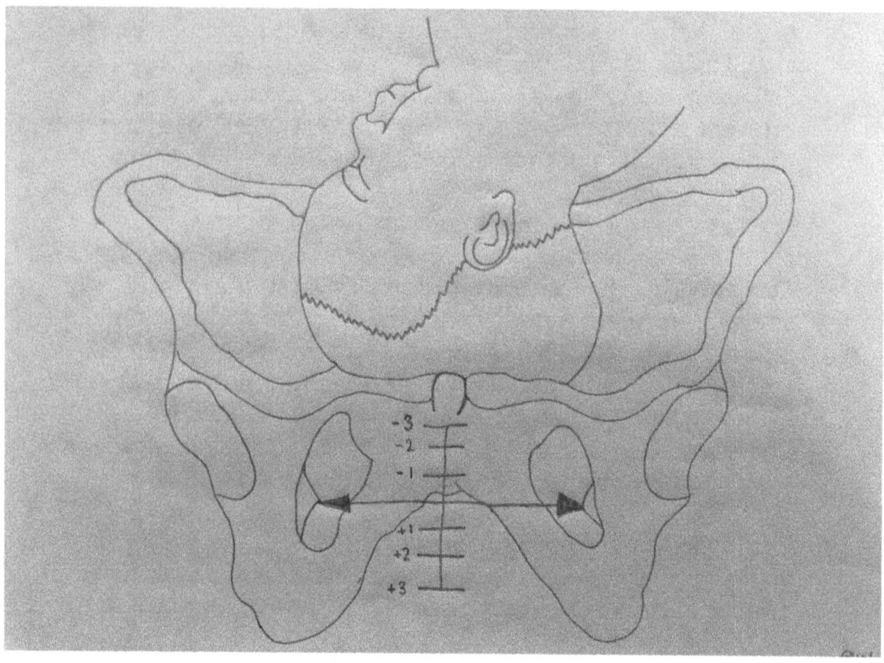

By using the orgasmic template, the symmetry of the sex hormones released will be released as your cervix dilates in ready-
ment for the journey through the birth canal, which, in turn
can be complemented by the convulsant reaction to pleasure
your within your vaginal walls and lower pelvis, as you will
most effectively form a layer of pleasure where there would be
only contraction constriction and pain.

It's a synergy, like a dance if you can visualise as you experience contraction, so too you experience a wave of the sensation of calm, then the sensation of warmth and pleasure. You
have a new layer of comfort and pleasure which moved with
you through the contracting layers of muscle the relief, as the
hormones released and increased through the space of sexual
arousal to compliment to the stages of labour.
The fusion is amplified, when you increase the release of sex
hormones at the same time the birthing hormones. The influence is greater. This is what I refer to as the orgasmic template.

If you study the science of orgasm familiarise yourself with
the layers, then learn the layers of childbirth we are mapping
the two together as the sequences of this text will show you,

then you can become one with the pain or discomfort and one with the pleasure. The two cannot co-exist.

The layers that mirror are.

1. Hormones - oxytocin, prolactin, and vasopressin cortisol

2. Movement contraction / Convulsant uterine and muscular contraction in orgasm. The pleasure spasms Exact same routine different context. Same areas of the body. Both effective.

3. Emotions Love vs Fear.
Love and fear are polarities. You cannot experience them both at the same time.
We are making sure you are on the right side of the equation. It's as simple as an equation when constructed this way. The motive is to increase pleasure in your own way. You are now educated in the science of orgasm will be educated in the science of birth when the two form together.

You have the layers here, you have the layers of birth within which the sequences of muscle movement are mirrored in birth and arousal to climax. At different degrees. The big O brings them together and use them to balance each other, neutralise discomfort and to provide you with your own form of natural pain relief as if nature had intended.

When you tune into the sensations of your body this makes a perfectly synonymous system. A concurrency. A cohesion.

Which instantly dissolves the pain. Oxytocin, prolactin and vasopressin all present in increasing measures alongside dopamine and serotonin and they all have their role to reduce pain and increase pleasure.

As if by a sliding scale. One decreases (pain) as Pleasure increases.

The next layer is to add into your preparation now you are aware of the sequence of labour and the timing of the release of the hormonal shifts and changes so you can time everything perfectly for your most cohesive and comfortable

experience.
When you are familiar with the layers of labour the enhancement and inclusion of intimacy as you go becomes easier.

Being aware of your own erogenous zones so you can use them frequently become more familiar with your body and the gentle sensations of pleasure you experience to give you sensations of leading to the birth of baby.

Your mental fixation becomes intently focussed on your body. Your breathing pacing each contraction with a firm flowing layer of arousal of excitement. Mentally, you are guided within to imagine baby moving through the birth baby birth canal. To move through the layers of labour feeling a sense of oneness with your body with your baby and with a growing sensation of sexual arousal beginning to build and maintain momentum though each contraction.

The sense of touch, when your body is naturally instinctively also holding a pattern of rejection to touch or the sensation of support when birthing because it has an instinctive build in motive to preserve energy. And assertion of boundary.

If this occurs similar to when you see the Movies when women are birthing, they scream, cuss and resentment of their partners. There is a better way to vent and tune your energy, it is more resourceful and more efficient to use arousal, to breathe baby down and to fixate and centralise on love.

There is a better way. That's to manage your energy inside and as you work through these pages the answers will ensue.

Beyond your waters breaking penetration is not advised, but there are so many other ways to induce arousal and stimulate pleasure. Without risking infection.

For example, clitoral stimulation massaging the perinium massaging the vaginal opening. Each act is an act of relaxation and arousal to incite pleasure and increase the release of the endorphins and oxytocin. For the intention of increasing comfort filling the void where pain could sit with pleasure. The two cannot co-exist in the central nervous system. Your partner can be involved where you are birthing singularly you can evoke your own sensations.

As labour progresses stage two, where contractions increase in gravity you have moments of pause five minutes or so, this is the window for pleasure to build so that when the contractions start, they are balanced with what has the potential to be a building orgasm.

Your ability to merge the orgasmic template at the exact moments you require it. The waves of contraction in labour meeting with the release of endorphins and the waves of pleasure sensations mirrored in the body.

The building release of hormones as tiem progresses through the labouring journey are your points of potential in maximising the cohesion For the most beneficial utilisation of the hormonal chemical load being effectively timed to spread merge in harmony at the exacting times you require.

The more functionally potent the contractions will be when your body is moving with them, so to contract, the muscles in your uterus tightening and moving baby through the birth canal and the sensation of release and pleasure as you do.
The reality is the exact same movement and contraction, BUT with a simultaneous layer of the chemical relaxation building within as a response to arousal, to relaxation to calm and to ongoing stimulation and the use of your clitoris for the one aim possibly its originally intended aim.

When you orgasm, you convulse, you stretch, the release of the hormones – serotonin, dopamine, oxytocin, vasopressin, it's a synonymous movement brought about by the timed sequence and release of the exact biochemical mix to supplement the movement and flow required of the body in labour. Supported, enhanced and even more so when working in harmony with the synergy within the big O to overcome the pain sensations by reducing the pain, flooding the senses with pleasure chemistry, actively supporting and supplementing the movement of flow that is labour.

A literal Mexican wave of muscular contraction, if you imagine a layer of movement in labour and then surround this with a layer of arousal induced chemistry which naturally reduces pain it doesnt oppose pain it simply overrides it.

When you are labouring your body contracts alone, as a reflex. It's encumbered by a layer of tension and discomfort. Which comes from two places, our thoughts fears and perceptible tensions and our resistance to the natural flow.
When this layer is reduced and becomes a layer of pleasure supplemented by the release of oxytocin, dopamine, serotonin, vasopressin and accompanying hormones, enhanced by the sensation of relaxation, combined with arousal there is a very powerful combination.

The new cohesion forms a unity mind, body, baby all working in harmony. And your ability to control and choreograph this process is becoming stronger the more you learn about the cohesion.
It's a synergy.
A symphony.

Its makes sense. Orgasms are possible, and you can use them, especially when you time it right. The knowing how to time it will come with faith and exploration. Knowing your body its intricacies its idiosyncracies, having faith in your body, your femininity and your confidence and acceptance of self-pleasure when in labour.

Now you can accept this you are 90% there.

Now you know, The cycle of arousal. What an orgasm is the stages how to make them, how to harness them, The female sexual body. So now you know, and can identify What an orgasm is, The stages of orgasm, The layers and how they can translate into the stages of child birth and it actually makes sense when it's overlayed.

Thy types of orgasm, an introduction to your body, and the places you can excite to make that happen and how to make them happen. Your uterus. It's intricate structure, and the emerging purpose for orgasmic template.

The stages of labour and what it means to overlay the orgasmic template, through your birthing experience. The chemical sequences. How to orchestrate the synergy of your dynamic organic structures and sequences, and how it makes sense so you can use it. You are familiar with your uterus, its role function and form and your erogenous zones, places to try places to learn and places to love.

So now you know, and can identify What an orgasm is, The stages of orgasm, The layers and how they can translate into the stages of child birth and it actually makes sense when it is overlayed. Call it The orgasmic Template.

The types of orgasm, an introduction to your body, and the places you can make excite to make that happen and how to make them happen. Your uterus - It's intricate structure and the emerging purpose for the orgasmic template.
The stages of labour and what it means to overlay the orgasmic template, through your birthing experience and how to actually do this
So now you know what an orgasmic birth is, that they are possible, not just spontaneously but when you actually believe that they are possible, and that you can choose to. That you can use your body's own cycles to and chemical trail to overcome discomfort in labour. You are beginning to wrap your head around the possibility that it is an actual real life possibility more so than a joke, or a laughable notion. The sequence of orgasm and arousal, your homework to experiment different scenarios, mentally physically. Different ideas on how to climax experiments. The chemical sequences. How to orchestrate the synergy of your dynamic organic structures and sequences, and how it makes sense so you can use it. You are familiar with your uterus, its role function and form and your erogenous zones, places to try places to learn and places to love.

CHAPTER FOUR

Your Body

" When I touched her body I believed that she was a god in the
curves of her form I found the birth of man and the creation
of the world" Roman Payne

Your body in fascinating detail. It's a miracle. Living breathing walking talking miracle We don't celebrate it enough - we
don't celebrate our bodies enough. They wake up, our heart
beats, we breathe we ourselves were formed from a single egg
and grew in our mother's womb. You are growing a miracle.
Every time we scuff our body it heals. Our bones heal and re
grow. Your body is a constantly repairing and replenishing
itself all the time and in in pregnancy it is magnified and
directed. What makes the most difference is the emotional
resonance you are carrying within you to expediate healing
and to experience healing. Have you heard people say that
after they have given birth, they forget the pain of childbirth.
Like it evaporates. If it didn't you might not do it again so it's
the natural ordinance of life.

What your body is capable of is unknown until it is tested.
People do iron man, run 100 mile ultra marathons and that is
just one single thing in the degree of endurance human body
is capable of. Do they think of the pain they will endure while
on an ultra-run … no!
They live for the run. And they wear good socks to avoid getting blisters. They plan for it. As you are now.

When you think about the potential your body has, childbirth
isn't such a great expectation. With the addition of the Big O
and everything that has been revealed so far it makes great
sense that you would have everything you needed already to
precede the birth itself and now you are learning to use it.

*You have everything you need inside to birth your baby. Nature
gave it to you.*

To make childbirth comfortable and to guide and push your baby through the birth canal as comfortable and efficiently as possible isn't a huge expectation.

The greatest task is to maintain calm, clarity and composure to allow for the body to progress within the security of the space to birth, you are in focused solely on one task to birth you baby.

The main three main concepts to grasp here are –

Calm. Using relaxation and fixation techniques

Confident – whatever your knowledge or your birth choices are, own them because. You embody a different level of confidence or faith when you own something. It's such a different determination or intention. It's a hue of grace when it's your choice you wear it proudly. You have a very different resonance. A sense of intactness. When you own the orgasmic template it works for you.

Control – When you are calm, you are in control of your immediate sensory perception of your environment. When you are in tune with your body in a level of calmness that is likened to meditation, you can pace your body to calm. Even your blood pressure.
You can control your thoughts, your response to the environmental changes around you. The people around you and to changing conditions. You can control how you perceive the world around you your actions.

Climax - Bringing the three together. Being calm, confident and in control of your mind and body, your thoughts. And use them in the direction of your choosing to experience pleasure and reduce pain.

Points of control and similarity in all birth practices.

1. Reduce stressors.

2. Include a central point of focus

3. Relaxation techniques – Including visualisation, hypnosis, and arousal.

Here once again you integrate all 3 and include number 4.

Your body has manufactured an entire life support system for your baby and you as its host. You have a unique life support system within you a life growth system. Fully engineered and perfected by you, without thought. Without conscious design. Or without intervention. You just are it. You just are. Including your ability to induce pain relieving hormones and biochemical mix, by simply including one simple addition. Believing the orgasmic template, that the clitoris is womans natural pain relieving centre where she can manage her pain in the most challenging of times and enjoy the sensation of owning that as a new found truth.

In birthing babies, the most amazing organ is your Uterus.

 In the Big O it is very closely followed by the clitoris.

The difference being that the clitoris has no role in fertility. You can make a baby without one. It's more enjoyable with one.

You are phenomenal.
A secure unit of absolutely everything, life support for your baby so it can grow and it can develop and thrive.
Your uterus and placenta provides the actual moment by moment conversion and calculation of everything that baby needs, bringing goodness in and taking waste away to a exact-ing changing formula.

In the external environment, how many machines does it take to keep that role fulfilled when your body can do it all within itself. The intelligence of your body is phenomenal. You do that. Without even thinking. It can do so with the chemical load of orgasm to be aligned with pain relief also. When you are unconsciously weighing out milk formula ... and how much science it takes to engineer to formula we buy, your body does that. Just by its ultra-design of baby after birth it naturally adjust the formulaic components of your milk perfectly for baby. You are that in tune. And it does this in Utero for the full 9 months.

Everything your baby needs is provided. Just like for you when you were in the womb.

Then look at the clitoris.

What is its purpose, pure pleasure.

It has one role.

Pleasure, to induce a biochemical shift in the body.

Repeatedly, So its role in childbirth must be just so. To acti-vate the pleasure centres, and reduce pain. To literally flush the sensation of pain from the body. Allow it to do what its naturally designed to do. In one completely natural act.

So, we can instead assume that it can be a pleasurable experi-ence. And learning how to refine your attention. Direct your thoughts, and energy into what supports your body.

The Mind body connection

A paradigm simplifies the interaction which will define your greatest life choices.

You can use the chain of interaction in any of the three routes. For example.

This book is using your MIND by being in your ENVIRON-EMNT to influence your BODY and it works by using your thoughts to change the resonance of your body.

Influence your environment by making choices differently to how you would have made them before and you are strength-ened in resolve and are more educated.

You are more educated so less swayed by the environment and therefore have more traction to influence the environment.

This is empowerment. You are more able to move the situation to your advantage and favour, because you have a stronger foothold of knowledge than you did before.

That becomes a bed of faith.

You choose the way your mind influences your body and you choose how your environment works for you the interaction between all 3 is more harmonious.

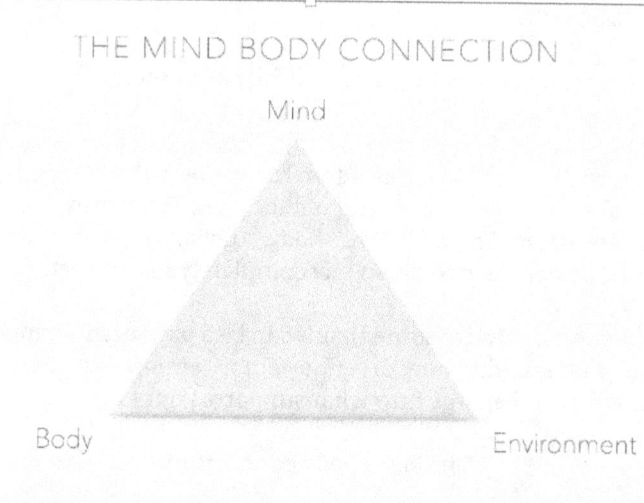

Mind

There are many, known medical professionals Doctors who have identified a deep connection between our thoughts and our bodies health, and our experience of life. The thought leaders in this spectrum include. Louise Hay, Candace Pert who looked into the emotional effect on molecular structures,

Bruce Lipton in the biology of belief who has the essence of the interaction between thoughts and cells being. Greg Braden and the Divine matrix the interconnectedness for the basic principal thoughts creating things amplified by feeling. Hidden messages of water Masaru Emoto - a book which brought to life actual pictural evidence the influence on intention words onto the frozen water.

The words love and gratitude made the crystalline structure very beautiful intricately woven crystalline structures actual symmetrical form so beautiful.
Clean and crisp and organised, elegant, and refined. And words hate and fear made the crystalline structures deformed and mutated, harsh, and asymmetrical.

This being true then the resonance of our cellular structure being water is heavily influenced by the components of communication that occurs within and around us what we say what we do, what we think.

We literally absorb it from the environment around us. Until like you are now. Knowledge changes our beliefs, they turn and strengthen so you are less influenced by the environmental influences.

And what begins to resonate with you as you are moving forward, changes. When you are confident in your choices you own them you move differently you feel differently and owning your choice to your the orgasmic template requires acceptance and inclusion.

We have filters which develope and evolve through life. And can choose what we allow ourselves to accept as true for us or not.
You can choose, to allow helpful influences inside and to allow unhelpful influences wash over you like water off a ducks back.

Like teflon.

For example

When baby is 8 weeks old you might choose to inoculate it from certain illnesses you can inoculate yourself from unhelpful influences by building resistance. By building strength consider supportive beliefs as the antibodies. Built to strengthen and secure your immunity to ... whatever is the unhelpful influence. Instead, what you will do is strengthen your core beliefs just like your body building muscle. You will strengthen your beliefs and your bubble, so unhelpful influences, actually, like water of a ducks back, roll away, without permeating the surface rather than using vital energy to sift through them. You will just know what is right for you and that is what birthing babies as a journey enables you to do. Almost effortless because as your beliefs strengthen the hue strengthens, like a layer of support around you invisibly and within you incubating you, as well as inoculating you from the perceptions that would lower your perceptions and incite fear.

Belief by osmosis is a given in life, it happens, thought now you are aware you can choose. And as you're building your hue, a hue of acceptance coherence adn intactness. It will work for you. The thoughts we have are instruction to our cells the words we use are instructions to our cells. It influences our resonance so listening to birthing babies and absorbing this book will only add helpful influences supportive layer of consciousness that can become you without effort. That's the value. Education changes the perception of what you believe, and as you reason through education the big O becomes more acceptable. More possible, more plausible, and once again something that you cannot not do.
In education, there see this as a high return on investment of time. Because it can't not become you in some way. It moves you.

Into being, something more capable more competent and stronger to the extent you believe it will so go all in. And to find value for you within you so long as you allow it to.

When you imagine the influence of the vibrational load of your thoughts on the composition of your body it makes sense to be kind to yourself to encapsulate love. Once again the over-riding premise is: Our thoughts influence our bodies and we can change that. Easily. Love feels better than hate. Go with that. There is no argument no reason that you can present that that is not so. That does not mean that you cannot assert yourself calmly and confidently.

When doing 1:1 sessions with clients. I include a component in the script a suggestion that they can communicate in a calm and diplomatic way. To take pause, breathe and then communicate what they were intending, not what they were expected to communicate not what they think they should communicate. But what they actually intended to communicate.

Just by being aware. And then making new choices. Learning new concepts. Broadening your perspective.

Chemically: When the contents of your mind are reflected and resonated in your body. In the context of childbirth. You are choosing to change the way you perceived childbirth by learning new ways to make it easier. More comfortable. You have more control. To change your perceptions of what is possible.

Your mind at ease will place your body at ease so the reflexes and stimulation will be able to flow and allow the secretion of oxytocin and progression of labour. In the Big O the correlations and synergy between the biochemical structure. And you.

Your body is listening to your thoughts, fears, known and unknown. It's also listening the reassurances and the inclusion of joy and the expansion of possibility and the chemical load of our bodies is reflected from our minds. Give your self permission to succeed and allow the orgasmic template to ork for you and it will. Your body and mind will support you.

Your body was designed to grow nurture and birth a baby centuries ago babies were birthed in the woods, alone.

At these times there were very few demands on life and the main survival challenges were to eat and hunt, and safety from external predators. It was clear what was a threat and what was not. Now our sensory environment contains so much which we believe is good for us but is not always the case. Our nervous system is confused by the amount of stimulation that is available to us.

Your chemical load is different now. The chemical hormonal load is consequential to the many stimuli from our environment from interactions in our everyday life.

So, tuning out of the noise news, the demands of everyday life, the noise of the environment, the noise of the digital devices even when they are quiet, the noise of the radio, and tune into your body.

To allow the birth process to progress birth and allow for the opening of the cervix, contraction of the uterine muscles all led by baby's desire to breath and the first kick response. Your body is linked to your thoughts so mind and body work in harmony.

Your environment: includes, actions behaviours, and also physical complication such as breach positioning and placenta positioning these are idiosyncrasies that can factor into birth planning and the process of birth however you can still control your experience of birth. Environment includes professionals and decisions about birth planning. The places and spaces around you. What you put in your body. The places you spend time - If you listen to fearful, judgemental people you will experience fearful thoughts, and the heaviness of the burden of their judgements. Though if you listen to the feelings of being calm confident and in control. Then you will experience being calm confident and in control. When you accept that your birthing choices are deeply personal and respected as such and build a number of reasons why it's important to you.INSIDE. With out sharing your reasons, they build a hue of intactness that becomes unshakable. The more you strengthen it the more you become it.

When you are literally feeding your mind with stories of woe and risk this is what is nourishing your mind. Change that. Learn something different. When you absorb the content of this book, and audios even the birthing baby's course. It will inoculate you into a bubble of your own strength of thought and belief so no matter what the environmental circumstances are, you are stronger within to both manage the environment either change it or work with it or form a new plan. You will have their knowledge working within you for you will have the sentiment of everything you didn't realise working for you within. It inoculates you without you even thinking. You build a confidence, once again it's the hue. The hue is around you and it is a strength and intactness. You accept what you are doing as right for you, even if it's different, or controversial.

As you listen as you live and as you learn it all becomes forward. It all becomes you and you become strong. That is the hue.

Pain versus Discomfort

Pain and discomfort - The strangest paradox is that pain is amplified by the tension in your mind through to your body in a way that causes the neurological impulses in the body creating tension and the tension causes constriction which causes pain. Because fear causes constriction. It calls the body to turn into fight or flight, mode of preservation of energy and causes constriction of the flow of blood to the muscles at the very basic level. To literally preserve life. But when it is misplaced, the primal instinct is triggered.

The constriction, is to preserve of life, your body is perceiving a threat on some level, even a minor trigger and instinctively withdrawing within to preserve the vital organs. To prolong life. In a primal way. As if the threat is a primal threat when in fact it may be triggered by a medical instrument tray or something so very small that is very innocuous in reality.

To overcome this, and to resolve the inappropriate fears and anxieties naturally caused by the response to the environmental cues around us, the relaxation sessions within this books appendix are very potent. To desensitise you to the cues in your environment that have unnecessary emotional attachments, ones that you wouldnt even be aware of until

you were in the moment.
Ones that do not serve you.

So to build your confidence in birthing baby to increase the flow in your body and to feel less fear, because your fear sensor has been re set. As a natural consequence the risk of intervention and the risk of problematic labour complications is reduced as much as you possibly can. Some situations always would remain out side of our control and there is always the potential for a need for medical or surgical intervention but you are doing whatever you can to reduce those possiblities and ensure a calm confident birth with increased comfort and a more coherent version of you.

So when you take it back to basics.

The potential that you think pain into being to some degree. Is helpful because then you can unthink it.

Not in it's entirety, but so you have mechanisms here that will enable you to reduce the sensation of pain.
To mentally overcome them by changing your thoughts and perceptions, influencing the biochemical flow of your body to improve your experience of birth.

The reduction of the sensation of pain is brought about by the balancing of the sensations within your mind as to the meaning of the pain.

Triggers for pain, often pain is a response to that something has changed something is different to divert your attention to the place in which you experience discomfort.

The signals though neurotransmitters alerting to movement and change therefore indicating an unknown and that something is different.

When the signal causes tension this slows the progression of the fergusson reflexive impulses chemically be reducing the amount of oxytocin produced and increasing the amount of adrenaline the stress hormones such as cortisol which inhibit the production and uptake of oxytocin and slow the progression of labour.

The Aim – The Three C's

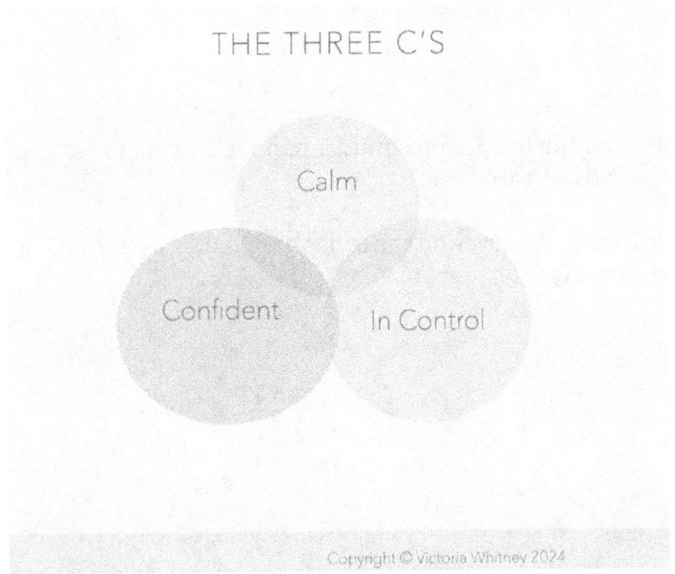

To be calm confident and in control to allow you to birth the way you choose and feel comfortable including the fourth C Climax.

The role of the hormones.

We have an autonomic nervous system is a component of the peripheral nervous system regulating involuntary responses such as heart rate, blood pressure, respiration, digestion and circulation. There are two branches of the Autonomic nervous system - Sympathetic and parasympathetic. Parasympathetic nervous system. Is an expansive state of attention wellbeing and flow of the attention and systems within your body circulating health and wellbeing and underpinning a greater sense of calm. You are relaxed and calm. Also Known as type B behaviour warm hands slow breath. Sympathetic nervous arousal is the sense of type A behaviour stress state fight or flight where the body is on constant alert. In which the blood flow is constricted and the body is less efficient. Sympathetic nervous arousal is symptomatic of fear based thoughts and triggers. When fear causes constriction.

It calls the body to turn into fight or flight and causes constriction of the flow of blood to the muscles at the very basic level.

With the aim to be calm confident and in control to reduce fears and increase flow.

One causes constriction the other has greater flow. And we can simplify it once more.

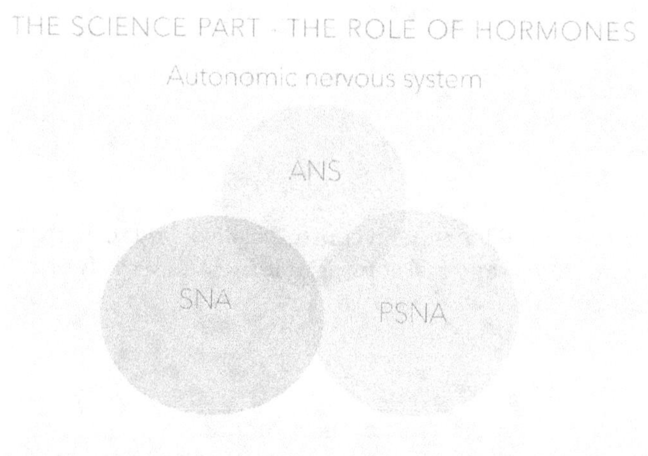

Faith VS FEAR.

Faith is born from fear and the two cannot co-exist simultaneously in the human nervous system. Much the same as pain and pleasure. The fear tension pain paradigm, can be reversed as calm comfort and flow .

The reverse of constriction is to alleviate the fears and bring within the sense of calm confidence and the application of helpful mechanisms of thought which will reduce the sensation of pain while keeping the functional purposes of pain as an instinctive response to the sensations of change within the body.

You need to feel pain when it is important.

If you experience cramping and bleeding it's important to instinctively calmly seek and follow medical advice.

Pain has purpose. But when pain is caused by anxiety and fear you can do more to overcome it by remaining calm confident and in control.

A paradigm explained is the relativity of a number of polarities, usually three which interconnect and can be inverted to bring about solution. It's formed from mathematics but basically, it's the solution to a problem.
When the fear amplifies the discomfort into pain causing tension. In the absence of fear and the presence of knowledge you are able to remain calm. Education gives you new insights and fresh filters integrated so you feel less fear because you are aware they are kwons not unknowns.

You can be more confident adn feel less fear, feel more self assured.

More centred more coherent and more intact.

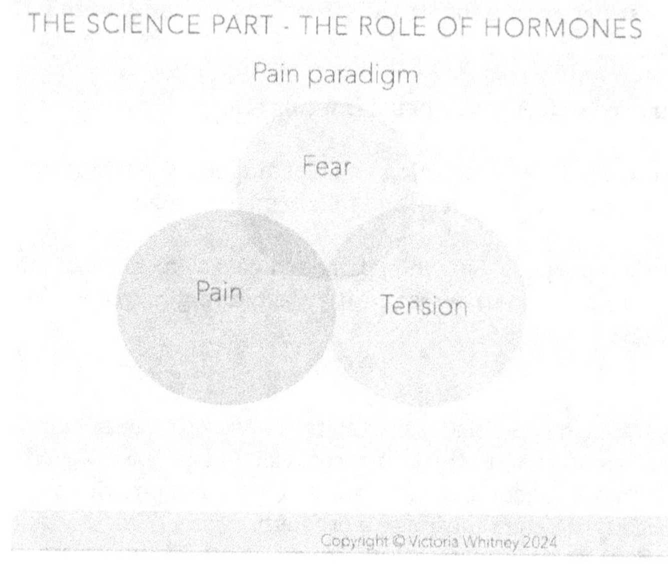

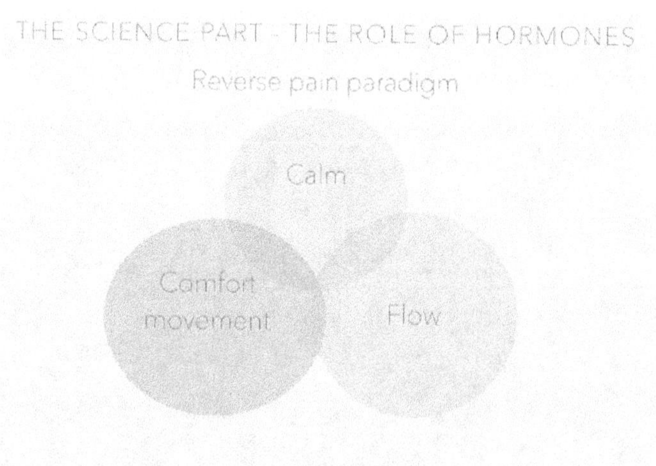

Everyone has their own pain threshold.

And it can change.

Your educated filters change the relationship you have with

pain and the fears, and the experience of discomfort. That's caused the tension and caused the pain in the first place, so you will by - product of reading this book alter your level of pain. And the more you work with the concepts the pain will be reduced.

Does this mean you can't use pain medication.
 Hell no. It's just an addition.

It's your choice.

Some people do for various reasons, chemicals, and baby, for their own strength everyone's birth choices are personal and there is a no judgement. It's your choice. This is just the space where you can define your own journey.

to make your own choices and define your own path. You can assert your choices and own your choices because you are educated and confident in those assertions.

Everything you need inside to be calm confident and in control is already within you.

Its your choice. If you choose to use medication then own it, as a choice. Thats what makes the difference.
Then you are stronger in your assertion.

I remain very much pro-choice in the moment. And present the possibility that childbirth can be comfortable and pleasurable even without medication.

Now you have a grasp of the concept of pain in the body and how stress, and tension influences the biochemical load in our body there are several ways to influence thi, to overcome it. And own your own experience of pain.

The Pain pleasure paradigm.

The simplicity, of the pain pleasure paradigm.
Reverse pain paradigm when, relaxation is present there is an anomaly which enables the fear to disperse and for relaxation to be present. When this is so. It's possible for the theory of pain pleasure to be conceived. When taken to the extreme the pleasure as an enhancement of calm, you can significantly reduce the degree of pain experienced because pain and pleasure cannot coexist at the same time. So, the pleasure

overtakes the sensation or concept of pain first in the body then in the mind. They then work as a synchronous flow of hormones and sensations which enhance the pleasure and maintain the sensations for longer. The most efficient meaning for a woman is that you have the ability to experience multiple sensations of climax with an expedient recovery time between. So that you can begin again to maintain the maximum sensation of pain relief.

The science of pain and pleasure is that you can't physically experience the experience of pain when you feel pleasure much like you can experience the feeling of fear when you feel love.

It's so efficient. And you need to look nowhere but inside to access it. It already there within you. It is organic pain relief Harel's (2007) study on sexual birth experiences demonstrated a trend of the use of clitoral stimulation as analgesia within orgasmic birth experiences. One of the participants of the study recalled that the only way she coped with the pain was through masturbation, utilising her sexuality to birth her baby (Harel, 2007).

The science of pain and pleasure is that you can't physically experience the experience of pain when you feel pleasure. Much like you can't experience the feeling of fear when you feel love. The two are polarities and it's as if you can switch them over, the sensation of contraction being a similar experience to the internal contractions you experience when you climax, it's the simple shift in magnitude and perspective.

So the climactic sensations begin to become a version of contraction when you stimulate them just at the right time, through the space between contraction, the contraction can become climactic, so the expansion is the sense you experience along with the contraction to increase the flow of the waves of contraction progressing baby through the birth canal as well as the sense of pleasure incited when you experience the sensation of arousal building to climax .

Contraction expansion, ripples like waves of peristeletic waves of pain or waves of pleasure. The synergy of the two interwoven natural instinctive flows becomes apparent. And make sense. And the polarity transition starts in your mind by seeing the possibility for it.

Pain versus Discomfort

Different people have different sensations of pain and very different threshold. But to use arousal, to manifest pain relief.

So, when you take it back to basics. Relaxation reduces the sensation of pain because the tension is reduced. The tension brought about the pre- conception and the fear of the pain makes the pain worse so the then reducing this to discomfort it makes it very simple and very effective to reduce. When you think about it. The pain becomes discomfort because the notion of pain does not exist. The discomfort and movement are the purpose of the electrical impulses in the body, the cellular purpose brought it into the flow of rhythmic muscular contractions are purposed by movement and flow. There was never a preconditioned intervention in nature which brought the theory of existence of pain, simply discomfort and movement. Only the ego of man or woman which brought the ignorance of what the body is capable of and what the body is doing.

The pain triggers fear of what the pain is. But the fear is of the unknown. Fear in labour is known. The quantity is known as to what it is once it is established that you are labouring. The pain causes a fear cycle. When you tune into your body and work with the fundamental controls. The fear is less because you are aware that the pain is a known and you can work with a known quantity. You can work easily with a known quantity and establish confidence to welcome the flow of contractions as they encourage you to work with them, to relax breathe and, and encourage the release of hormones, by relaxing into your body relaxing into a rhythm of releasing tensions and working with the orgasmic template.

Points of control and similarity in all birth practices.
They all include the following.

1. Reduce stressors

2. Include a central point of focus

3. Relaxation techniques – Including visualisation, hypnosis and arousal.

Birthing babies with the big O is to bring about an ability in a woman to manage her own level of comfort with unknown benefits to her own body and mind and that of her baby. By increasing the degree of pleasure. By overlaying the orgasmic template. And accepting that it is possible. Integrating it into their birthing practices.

Very simply

Arousal in childbirth enables a bypass, disperses the tension, eliminates the tension, Increases the expansion and flooding of pleasure hormones through the receptors literally flushes the sensation of pain with pleasure.

You are relaxed and the tension is an impulse of enjoyment and waves of pleasure, which mirror the waves of contraction. They work together in taking two completely natural instinctual excitements of the nervous system which have very different intentions and end points and allowing them to work in harmony. To become uniform. To merge and correlate. They are the same purpose but to bring them together is one of nature's greatest discoveries, especially for women. Perhaps this is the original purpose for the clitoris in its formation with its one unique purpose, as a source of pleasure.

It increases the emission of oxytocin and oxytocin is the expander of the sensations of pleasure (remember a 200 times Magnification on your morning coffee) increase the body relaxes and the natural peristaltic waves that occur as contraction, but also as the rythmic pulsations of climactic pleasure they are mirrored with two different purposes, but in harmony work together the orgasmic waves of pleasure that ripple through your body when you reach climax are simultaneously mirrored to the peristalticwaves of motion which move baby through the birth canal. Simply on a different scale.

Fear and excitement are both states of arousal.

Both with very similar biochemical makeups - but very different interpretations and motives and consequences. They are translated by the mind as to determine which is which. Through the surveying of billions of sensory cues.

Though sometimes they become confused. Give yourself permission to be excited. When the sensory cues have different meanings they become different in response.

Calm – relaxation flow.

This comes after the waves of orgasmic pleasure and the relaxation follows very gently. Even though you are aroused it's a different type of arousal. Which requires the sensation of centredness. Rather than the raw heated erotic passion. It will feel, sense more primal, with a maternal hue, and vein of purity and love for the pursuit of comfort and ease.

As we engage in self pleasure the nervous system becomes excited, excited into arousal and engorgement of the sexual organs.

Fight or flight and panic will inhibit this, it encourages the release of cortisol which inhibits the production of oxytocin. And the entirety of the pain relieving sensations beneficial to the body is paused until the cortisol secretion is overcome.

Sexual arousal is different it causes and increase in heart rate and increases the production of beta endorphin oxytocin and prolactin and vasopressin.

Oestrogen and testosterone are all increased enabling the body to relax and experience multiple sensations of ripples of orgasmic waves of pleasure through each cell fibre. Intensely. The more intensely, the more available parasympathetic nervous arousal is to the woman. In simple terms when she is calm confident and in control. Enough also to channel the excitement into her given task.

When it's so vital to stay calm, confident and in control, not just the I'm in control swoop in and save the day calm, but a deep sense of safety and awareness of the flow of life.

Fear causes the muscles in the body to constrict and reduces the flexibility of the muscles fibres which are required for the transition of baby through the birth canal comfortably and smoothly. In turn this will cause the sensations of pain to be optimised. Something to be avoided. Tension causes pain and restricts flow. Calm relaxation, trust and a sense of safety causes flexibility malleability and an increases flow.

Psychologically, pain can be learned out, so the fear isn't present. There is certainty there will be discomfort. But you can reduce it, becomes your new truth, so the fear loosens and loosens each time you remind yourself that it can be different, and you endeavour to continue to learn how. There does exist a continuum, a pleasure-pain continuum and orgasm as analgesia. Surprisingly Dick-Read (2004) highlighted the fear of pain as the biggest disturbance to the natural course of labour. Tension as a cause of pain is associated with sphincter law, with involuntary sphincter muscles being inhibited by fear and environmental stress, with birth working best in privacy. Or with inoculation and building of confidence to occupy the personal space without fear or judgement (requiring acceptance of the whole premise of the capability of a woman to birth)

The body's response during sexual activity reflects this, where potential pleasure can be perceived as pain depending on the sensitivity of the sexual partner and the emotional participation of the female. In birth, this concept applies to rectal, cervical, and vaginal sphincters, which function best in an atmosphere of privacy, amd safety, comfort trust and harmony. And they begin restricting, if levels of adrenaline in the bloodstream increase.

Have you ever been unable to pee because there were people in the cubicles outside.

It is like relaxation, gentle music, visualisation, all contribute to the fixation of calm as an attention. To normalise the sensation of calm in places where environmental triggers may precede fear and thereby normalise them with the appearance of safety inside. And relay the sensation of calm as the fixation of attention.

This hugely supports the proposition that both Birthing Babies and Birthing babies with the "Big O" Suggests. And can be over come using gentle relaxation and desensitisation techniques to normalise the clinical environments such that they no longer trigger the stress response.

In Birthing babies, the audio version there is a caesarean desensitisation script, a relaxation to overcome the fear of the clinical environment. To build the sense of familiarity and comfort even in environments that are particularly challenging.

Desensitisation is incredibly powerful, because it raises the familiarity of the space the woman is in on a primal level. Which makes it ok to be there she feels safe to birth. The very slight undertone of fear that could possibly act as an undercurrent and restrict relaxation without even conscious awareness, of what is triggering the anxiety undertone, that the source cannot be delineated but can be overcome through gentle suggestion to the contrary encouraging the space of trust and safety within the birthing room.

We can already concede that many of the barriers highlighted in many studies about the environment birth occurs in, in fact we often talk about the mind body connection and using arousal to match the natural progression of labour to diminish sensations of pain is one epic use of this but, to learn it is one thing to know it and to do it is another.

The concept the mind body connection works just so.

Simply becoming accustomed with the potential for orgasmic birth means you are beginning to move towards the reverse pain paradigm instead. When you compare the two you can see who they can naturally literally be re translated. Where the increase of the hormones Dopamine, serotonin and Oxytocin are all increased because the turn on the stimulus is present where your body and mind are working together. Chemically these looks like this, they are beautiful.

OXYTOCIN

The increasing these hormones is a DIRECT result of reducing stressors and increasing relaxation and the use of arousal to increase the sex hormones.

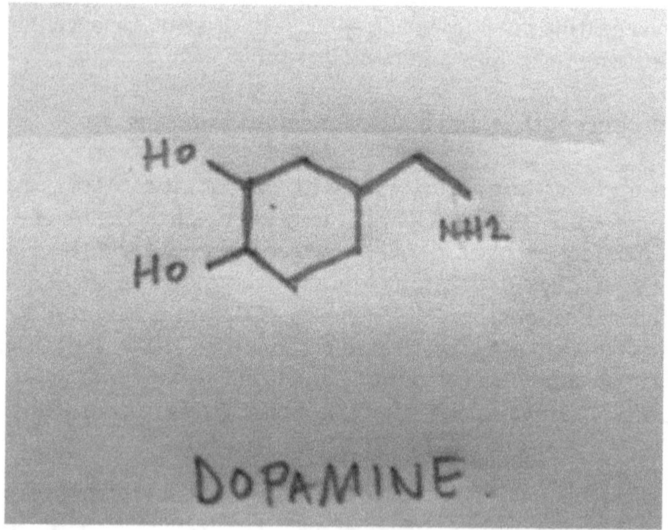

Fear vs Love – Pain vs pleasure

So to define, the relationship between Adrenaline and noradrenaline, as the amazing architecture of the hormones of birth and pleasure which also are present in fear and pain. The principle is when pleasure is enhanced, the emotional turn, or reflection to the chemical responses, hormonal releases, is enhanced. Increasing malleability rather than constricting. Contracting with pleasure, layered within the functional purpose of the contractions. When the muscular structures are filled with more pleasure hormones they are constructed differently than normal, even normal in labour. So they feel and behave differently.

The muscles move in peristaltic waves to bring baby through the birth canal, they are mirrored in orgasm when your body convulses. The arousal begins to excite the nervous system and produce the hormones which bring about the pain reversal. The increasing hue that comes from the sensation of arousal and build-up of the pleasure hormones, both in and out of labour give you a hue of well-being.

So you are less lucid to the sensations of pain, when contracting you are aroused. In very simple terms when you correlate the two concepts and bring it all together, it makes so much sense it is as if it was what nature would have intended in its origination.

Adrenaline hormones are released in response to stresses (for example, labour), triggering the 'fight or flight' response (Odent, 2009; Buckley, 2015). As in labour, adrenaline and noradrenaline levels also both rise with sexual arousal, peaking at orgasm (Exton et al, 1999). So they can be tuned into and moved into a different space and intention, being from pain and fear to pleasure and love. By education, and manipulation of the female form to increase sensations of pleasure and reduce pain.

Conditions for labour parallel those required for sexual intercourse, so it is simply a change in our minds.

With the potential for and magnitude of orgasm decreasing significantly when fear of performance is present, with privacy being both crucial in sexual relationships and birthing Fear being a hugely influential factor in the transition through birth and through performance in sexual intercourse. When you feel comfortable, familiar and have a degree of acceptance, your body responds with greater sensation, and pleasure. You have the space within to be able to be present because the thing you were fearing is less present you

have space in your mind to enjoy the things you love.
Fear diminishes and becomes a non thing.

Beta-endorphins are a group of opiate-like peptides released
from the pituitary gland in response to stress and pain, with
the same analgesic effects as exogenous opiates such as
pethidine (Buckley, 2015). High levels of endorphin release
have been described as inducing euphoric, orgasmic states
of pleasure (Bodnar, 2008; Veening and Barendregt, 2015),
acting as the body's natural pain relief in undisturbed labour
(Myles, 2014).

Although poorly understood, it is suggested that the role of
beta-endorphins in human sexual behaviour may parallel
its release during labour and birth, with high post-orgasmic
endorphin levels functioning to promote satisfaction and
bonding between sexual partners, reflective of the attachment effects between mother and baby.

In 2 studies with 10 women each, vaginal self-stimulation
significantly increased the threshold to detect and tolerate
painful finger compression but did not significantly affect
the threshold to detect innocuous tactile stimulation. The vaginal self-stimulation was applied with a specially designed
pressure transducer assembly to produce a report of pressure
or pleasure. In the first study, 6 of the women perceived the
vaginal stimulation as producing pleasure. During that condition, the pain tolerance threshold increased significantly
by 36.8% and the pain detection threshold increased significantly by 53%. A second study utilized other types of stimuli.
Vaginal self-stimulation perceived as pressure significantly
increased the pain tolerance threshold by 40.3% and the pain
detection threshold by 47.4%. In the second study, when
the vaginal stimulation was self-applied in a manner that
produced orgasm, the pain tolerance threshold and pain
detection threshold increased significantly by 74.6% and
106.7% respectively, while the tactile threshold remained
unaffected. A variety of control conditions, including various
types of distraction, did not significantly elevate pain or
tactile thresholds. We conclude that in women, vaginal self-
stimulation decreases pain sensitivity. When fear of pain is
present the production of oxytocin is diminished and therefore reduces the sensation of pleasure with a distraction fixation on an alternative.

————

This can be elevated through meditation, Hypnosis and self-led relaxation, so the fixation becomes a different point. As per Birthing babies – The Ultimate guide to Empowered birth. Overcoming the fears and preconceptions and judgements you have been pre-loaded with is also important. The acceptance you feel diminishes a sense of self consciousness. When you can justify your behaviour to your own mind, the benefits and the science of Orgasms enhancing your birth, is a much more effective and much more concentrated. So, you can confidently do it with efficacy and most importantly no shame.

The greatest barrier most will have in embracing the concept in reality bringing a differentiation as identified earlier in the book between sex and arousal in childbirth. Two very different purposes. Here we aren't clinicalising arousal we are acclimatising the mind where arousal is acceptable as is feminine empowerment in the birthing suite. Where you research read books such as Birthing babies by Victoria Whitney you are educated in the other side of childbirth the one that isn't publicised or made on TV the one where there is less drama even if emergent situations happen. The one where you are self-supporting and have faith and confidence.

One where you are comfortable confident even enough to self-pleasure in the birthing suite. The disparity becomes a distinction, when the distance between the two is measured and is corroborated, harmonised as each individual space within you as a woman is sacred. One arousal in child birth and two intimacy in the bedroom (or wherever else you choose). There becomes a convergence. You are one with many facets and these are two new facets that can bring great lasting harmony to yourself acceptance. Then the disparity falls away, and you can see a path where sexual arousal can perfectly coalesce to provide a very powerful birthing experience.

Imagine the greatest possible inclusion of two incredibly powerful forces of pain relief where you can experience birth as a scared space. Where you can independently influence the level of comfort you experience throughout. Where you are enough a one woman essence who can manage control and experience her own level of comfort from within.

Absorb the science and biochemistry of childbirth, combined with the synergy or labour in and climactic ebb and flow meeting and matching with the bio chemical and physical rhythm of birth and it becomes clear.

That one intense concept to grasp or perhaps true intention of our physical and chemical makeup from the origination was just this way, this is a huge turning point for the evolution of woman.

Back to the science - The relationship between Adrenaline and noradrenaline Adrenaline hormones are released in response to stresses (for example, labour), triggering the 'fight or flight' response (Odent, 2009; Buckley, 2015). As they do in labour, adrenaline and noradrenaline levels also both rise significantly with sexual arousal, peaking at orgasm (Exton et al, 1999). It's just a different turn, sexual arousal and nervous fear arousal. What happens commonly in labour is that the trigger of the adrenaline response is fear orientated. This can be changed. It's an essential component BUT it can be turned into a helpful sense of arousal to compliment and condition and control.

Conditions for labour parallel those required for sexual intercourse, so it is simply a turn on perspective. With the potential for and magnitude of orgasm decreasing significantly when fear of performance is present, with privacy being both crucial in sexual relationships and birthing Fear being a hugely influential factor in the transition through birth and also through performance in sexual intercourse. So you can formulate your birth plan to accommodate this. Make allowances such that you can feel confident on any environment using what you have learned.

When fear of pain is present the production of oxytocin is diminished and therefore reduces the sensation of pleasure with a distraction fixation on an alternative.

This can be elevated through hypnosis and guided relaxation, so the fixation becomes a different point. As per Birthing babies – The Ultimate guide to Empowered birth.

When this happens. Oxytocin eliminates stress hormones

flushing them out. Serotonin, it's role is to leave you with a general sense of uplifted wellbeing all around. Dopamine, the purpose of dopamine to provide pleasure satisfaction and motivation.

The actual orgasm itself is about 60 seconds of rhythmic contractions of the uterus vagina and clitoris and send a influx of oxytocin dopamine and serotonin through the whole body. Which lasts significantly longer.
During arousal dopamine levels are stable yet rapidly increase at orgasm then drop. The Dopamine - Prolactin response is different, as dopamine rises and peaks during orgasm it drops and prolactin begins to overtake it. Much is the response in birth when prolactin, oxytocin, dopamine and serotonin all build and peak as birth nears.
Coalescence of Climax and birth would naturally appear to be a near perfect organically ordinated combination. Pre ordained to increase the body's own ability to birth baby in a way that is comfortable, and with the essence of babies creation underpinning it.

Supported by childbirth activist Kitzinger (2012) reports that for many women there is a narrow separation between intense pleasure and pain, and that the sensations can often be bittersweet. Emerging neuroscientific evidence indicates clear similarities between the neurochemistry and neuro-physiology of the pain and pleasure systems (Leknes and Tracey, 2008; Moccia et al, 2018), and studies have illustrated the significance of the opioid and dopamine systems in modulating both pain and pleasure, with either sensation inhibiting the other (Wager et al, 2007; Leknes and Tracey, 2008). Suzanne Arms (1994) depicted this relationship as a paradox, suggesting that if fear can influence perceptions of pain and subsequently the course of labour, then alternatively anything that increases a woman's wellbeing, such as pleasure, will lessen her perception of pain. And enhance her wellbeing.

Turning perspective forward to arousal and climax. During excitement your vagina lengthens the vaginal cells begin to moisten the vagina. The clitoris expands and can even protrude outside of the labia. Levels of hormones serotonin, and dopamine increase your pupils dilate. (At just the time your that the relaxation of the vaginal and cervical walls would be of functional value)

Your Brain generates beta brain waves which are relatively low amplitude, but the fastest of the Brain waves. 15 – 40 cps. Cycles per second. Your senses are more alert to the fixation of the sensation of your body, the pleasure cycles and touch taste sense smell, and the pleasure of the sensations.

Stimulation activates the hippocampus and manages our memories sights and smells in the moment. The amygdala which governs sexual drive awakens they are communicated to the pre frontal cortex. The frontal cortex of the brain becomes aroused and can be centred fixated on the intention of calm comfortable birthing. Finally, the anterior cingulate cortex, which is thought to be involved in modulating pain, turns on.

The most striking point in the above data is the duality of the relationship between pain and pleasure. How the systems are so similar and interwoven that they can be mutually turned to overcome sensations of pain and experience a pleasurable birth in context. By using the mind, to influence the body and reconcile the environment within the space of them both. Centre the Points of control and similarity in all birth practices, reduce stressors, include a central point of focus to guide to intention of the nervous systems changes by using relaxation techniques including visualisation, hypnosis and arousal or a combination of all 3. To increase wellbeing, reduce the sensation of pain and accelerate healing.

Increasing the wellbeing within the mother naturally influences the wellbeing of the infant. When on a cellular level the infant is influenced just as the water crystals mentioned before, as you are calm baby is calm, even on its transition through the birth canal. At every point baby is tuned to your emotional state of calm, at all times you are cam confident and in control. You have the sensation of arousal and it is calm and measured, measured by your mind and harnessed with the purpose of birthing baby confidently calmly and with less pain.

Increasing the pleasure sensations means baby feels the sense of excitement, the sensations of joy and pleasure and the general sense of wellbeing which passes through your body when you are reducing stressors, using fixation and visualisation such as hypnosis, relaxation and arousal. Labour is less arduous, It becomes a rhythmic flow. The contractions are the same but your sensation is different. Imagine the influence on the general new-born health of your baby.

Apgar scores are an immediate evaluation of new-born health.. It is obtained by adding points (2, 1, or 0) for heart rate, respiratory effort, muscle tone, response to stimulation, and skin coloration; a score of ten represents the best possible condition. This is an immediate assessment of your babies health and wellbeing. They do not predict mortality as they can improve very quickly. If birth is long and arduous they can be lower. Or if there is a requirement for intervention they may be lower. As you can imagine. After a 20 hour working day you would be tired. If this 20 hour work day was graced with a space of rejuvenation and love, repeated rounds of the sensation of ultimate pleasure waves, faith and fixation on absolute love, intactness and an internal faith that everything good in you was working with you for you to achieve the days task you would likely feel less exhausted.

As would baby as your passenger. There is a parallel between the induction of stress on the body and lower health. That is fact.

Relaxation as an enhancement brought about by the relaxation and sense and strength of calm within the woman who births make sense. The use of arousal for pain relieving waves of hormones and biochemical inducement is helpful. Well being, being referred to baby through the entire process.

There are available guided relaxations at the rear of this book, and available to purchase via www.victoriawhitney.com/ onlinetraining

When you listen to a relaxation audio the greater health and well being that will prevail. Fears become transitory. There is a real truth in this. You can record the sessions at the rear of this book for your own personal use.

No matter how we reason out of it, no matter how we begin to embody the disquiet that is the opposition, the uprising and the denial of a latent truth. It isn't a statement of imposition of a belief, it is science. Saying that relaxation and the strength of fixation of attention on calm balance within the birthing woman brings greater health to the woman and the baby. That makes sense. That is truth and it is evident Birth Apgar scores higher when babies are born with hypnosis for child birth. It makes sense.

Calm mother calm baby, the physiological components laid out, it makes sense chemically, physically and environmentally no matter how much intervention is required. It is still possible. Because the influence is on your experience. Your body your attitude, your perspective.

So your focus changes and therefore yours and your babies experience of birth changes into something within your experience as something that you can control.

It is suggested that babies have better infant apgar scores following hypnosis and a shorter stage 1 labour [4] Whether this is a proven fact or simply a theory makes little difference in reality. I have seen many times when there is no statistical significance of benefits of uses of therapies. Yet had I recorded their effectiveness by asserting the same principles that I do routinely and applied from my back dated experience of statistical significance from Psychology training many years ago I would have likely found significance. The significance isn't that which is to provide a factual base for individuals to decide. There is a time when there is a requirement for this, but most often the actual faith that something is to effectively transition your thinking between the space of fear and faith is a leap. These leaps don't often have a basis of factual evidence because often it is too remarkable for us even to imagine as true.

Faith is immeasurable. If we did, we would be forced to believe in something greater than ourselves which is a leap in and of itself. That your body can defy what it has been taught and learned. That you have a natural inbuilt pain management system ready there, but we have been taught to fear it, like so many things that are good for us.

We are very much for proof, and empirical data. And sometimes to make something empirical sometimes limits its potential expansion because it is so definitive. When answers are sought, they are sought with purpose and when the purpose is exclusive, it is biased.

It is empirically clean but the perception will be based on the hypothesis of the outcome expected.

That is what studies do. They have parameters.

They cannot explain why the clitoris has only one role and that is pleasure they cannot empirically prove that its design was or was not to be utilised to be harnessed in childbirth to reduce pain.

They can measure the number of sensors and make qualitative assimilations of a number of women who achieve and succeed using a process and do not.

But if one woman believes it is possible then a woman can make that belief true. And experience her own perceptions of the already present proven facts and make them work to her own advantage. To bring about a birth not only graced with less pain but with pleasure instead. To bring about a combination of all the possibilities, of health of minimal pain of efficiency of labour of efficacy and confidence in making the choice to embrace the path or arousal to make her birth more comfortable. To embrace her own sexuality in a different way and retain the intensity and purity of sexual union with her partner as a separate and also sacred space. To differentiate and define herself within. To use her own mind, body connection and combination to make all work for her. Because she chose to command her mind and influence each and every cell with the grace of something good.

You can't measure the difference in someone's eyes when they have cleared a lifelong problem with numbers. You can ask questions to empirically prove the difference before and after. But to suggest that something does not work because it is not empirically tested can lead to ignorance of a great solution. It is the change in people's lives health and the equivalent in life changes that is evidence to me. And to them and that is why they return that is why they continue because it works. Make use of the visualisation techniques, time after time and notice how things change. It's the Hue. It's invisible but remarkably visible and it brings such great strength and fortitude. That is what resonates within you through your birthing journey.

And you can make it so. And believe that you can.

Now you know, The cycle of arousal. What an orgasm is the stages how to make the, how to harness them, The female sexual body. So now you know, and can identify, What an orgasm is, The stages of orgasm, The layers and how they can translate into the stages of child birth and it actually makes sense when it's overlayed.

The types of orgasm, an introduction to your body, and the places you can make excite to make that happen and how to make them happen.

Your uterus. It's intricate structure and the emerging purpose for the orgasmic template.

The stages of labour and what it means to overlay the orgasmic template, through your birthing experience. The chemical sequences, how to orchestrate the synergy of your dynamic organic structures and sequences, and how it makes sense so you can use it. You are familiar with your uterus, it's role function and form and your erogenous zones, places to try places to learn and places to love.

You know the intricate structure of your uterus, The pain pleasure paradigm, how to reverse pain sensations, how to breathe to pervade calm, the mind body connection, the purity of the origination of your physical makeup on a cellular level and how to influence this with each act thought word and deed. The construction, production and mixture of biochemical synergy that occurs in labour and orgasm, the orgasmic template overlaying birth.

CHAPTER FIVE

Labour

"Giving birth is an incredible act of nature and power." - Michele Obama.

It's show time .....

Traditionally the phases of labour are broken down into stages. As your progress can be measured and you will know where you are in relation to your babies birth.

STAGE ONE
First stage of labour

Common experiences will include.... Body heat will rise or drop. You will urge to empty bladder Hiccup or feel nauseated as your body begins to shift around the activity in your uterine muscles. At this time, you are aware that something is changing, and you will automatically know, so the sense of excitement the rush that comes as the onset or present of the birthing instinct is within your awareness. When you are aware of what it is you can move with it. When you are unsure if it is starting you become to confuse the rush wave with fear and that's unnecessary because it's your body telling you there is change. With education you are aware and there is less fear.

Your time to begin to become one with the birth of baby is now, the synergistic wave begins, your body will begin to contract and now is the time to feel a sense of warmth acceptance, of the movement and flow with which your body and baby will move in for the coming hours of the journey.
Bringing everything together so you are one woman birthing baby calmly confidently and with less pain.
You listen to your body, time the contractions the waves

of movement and stay present focussed. Listen to calming music, take a shower, be guided by instincts which show you the way to comfort.

The coalescence, choreography of Arousal and the stages of labour. You are harnessing the very peak performance of the endocrine system to support the synergy of birth.

The hormonal synergy and to meet each phase with strength. Use your natural pleasure centres to bring pleasure waves to inoculate your nervous system from the intensity of the pain that potentializes through labour.

As the baby moves through the birth canal and the vagina, your feel a sense of excitement and growing waves of climactic sensations, or orgasmic pleasure waves moving through each cell of your body. Is a helpful affirmation to use.

The sensations of pain become pleasure because you foresee them, and prelude them by building layers of biochemical synergy, to increase the chemical flow of the pleasure hormones so the sensation of pain is desensitised through fixation of attention, guided relaxation, orgasm, climax, and ongoing arousal. You are now familiar with the role of the clitoris as a purely purposed for pleasure in its origination. This is the time to use that purpose and include its participation in your labour to prelude the sensations of pain and to encourage more efficiency in labour. Building the layers of chemistry to produce a dimming sensation to the discomfort of contraction, so you feel the uterine contractions and are one with them, they come and they go, each one stronger and bringing you closer to birthing your baby though you are at one because you are breathing, you are calm, you are centred moving when you need to and you are using your clitoris and vagina, to increase your sensation of arousal throughout this time, to ease the discomfort in exactly the space that it exists and originates and you are merging the concept of birth and the precedent creation of the centres for pleasure as they were intended without shame. Centred within you pace the sensation of contraction and breathe pace the sensation of contraction massaging, vibrating however you choose, though you are in tune with the rawness by the symmetry and synergy and unification of orgasm and birth. Here is where you will feel everything begin to come together and everything will make sense.

The experiences you may feel at the onset of labour include. These aren't exclusive and there are many more. You will have the sense for the need to escape, possibly as a reverse flow of the baby's sensations to you. How, sometimes people suggest that you have personality changes when you are in pregnancy like you have waves of the soul of the baby. The waves of the personality of the baby. Much like when your body moves you towards the same space in you will feel that sense of urgency to escape though you could interpret this as baby is coming. And a desire to find a safe space to begin the process of labouring baby. Your sense of time will become distorted you will be so focussed and absorbed. Into the process. Like ultramarathon runners. The best ones I know do not check their watches. Do not check with time because they are so at one with the run that they just keep going it is as if it is another world to them, they are running. Therefore, the run has a life of its own. From start to finish they are running and the only thing that is of matter to them at that time is their run and being centred within the run. Not thinking how long is left or even putting one foot in front of the other they are just one whole running. They just keep going until they get to the end. You are birthing. Just like that. Consider this a birthing day. It's a birthday the babies first birthday that you are completely absorbed in. Your first birthday to baby. The one on all of which are built here after, and you stay calm confident and in control; Therefore, you are birthing and that is what you are doing. Time is for the midwives to monitor you, as your purpose is to birth and enjoy the breathing and centring and contraction of breathing of baby down, and then, the final moments of pushing. Is what you are doing. It's as if it's one of those times in your life when you will feel completely taken care of – it's as if as you move though the book and use the relaxation sessions, your mind is going ahead and making it so. That you are totally taken care of in all ways so that all you can do is stay centred. Everything in the world appears to stop.

Transition phase - shift to birthing breathing down.

You are breathing down into your abdomen.

You are breathing down the act of your breath and muscles working in this way will use your energy to push baby down.

Pushing the uterine muscles will further the progression of

labour by utilising the muscular movement to engage the muscles in the abdomen. It will also calm the impulses and bring order to the chaos of the movement of the stimulus which has began the progression of labour. It gives the energy and impulses direction, so you experience less of the random sensations. You are directing your attention and energy with each breath and the progression of labour will continue with your control of your breathing in a calm confident sensation will become you.

Abdominal breathing

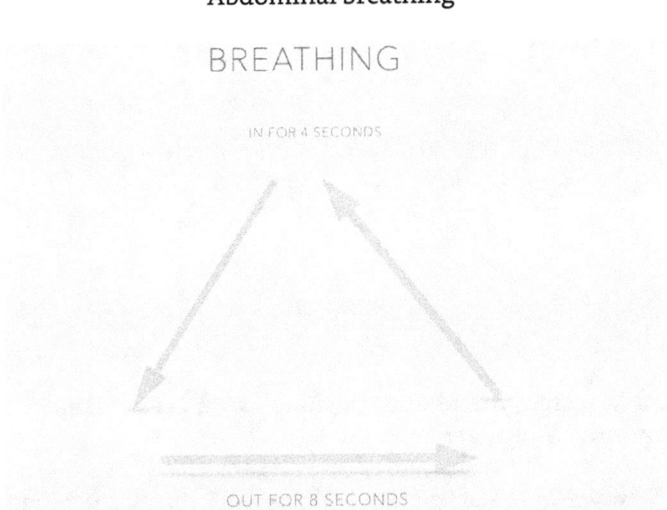

Deep breath in and a one to two ratio on the out breath -the outbreath twice as long as the in breath.

You can also include what is now become fashionable - box breathing.

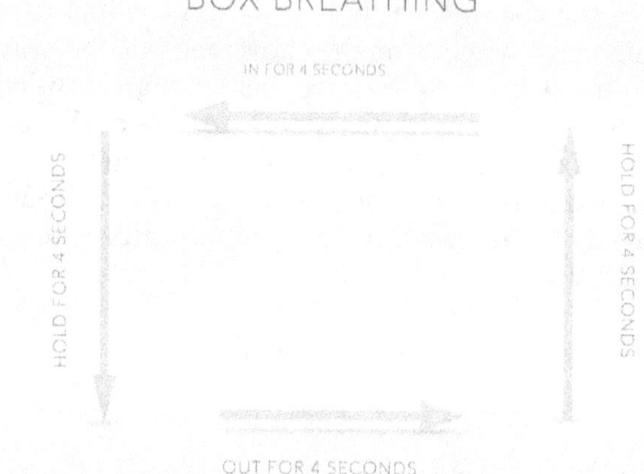

Breathe in for 4 seconds...hold for four seconds... breathe out for four seconds .....hold for four seconds.

PUSHING

At this point, you are not pushing – You are breathing the baby out. It is different.

The waves in the uterus are peristaltic waves – They become stronger, but they are no stronger than you. They are waves of movement with purpose like pulses. Any forced pushing hinders progress. When your body wants to push the energy of the push is very powerful and comes close to the end of labour. If you have ever felt the need to push and been asked to stop pushing when your body wants to push you will understand, though with these techniques you can refine and control the energy of the bodie's inclination to push by harnessing your focus into a breath this brings your attention and central nervous system to distribute the energy by giving it another purpose. With an overwhelming physical urge to push this will begin, the energy of the movement of the push, becomes focus on your breathing to maintain the energy of movement at your control.
In the breath it will feel more comfortable, breathe the pressure out. Very simply it gives it somewhere to go that is helpful and focussed and supports your body in birthing baby. With minimal distress. This protects your body from

unnecessary strain by giving more oxygen to the muscles in your body to flex and move as you are calm so are they as you trust and move with your breath so do, they. And the urges to push will be activated and progressed when they are necessary. Using breathing to control pushing. Oxygenates the muscles most importantly the perineum and will allow the perineum to be flexible because of the state of calm that pervades you. Pushing in the later stages of delivery being calmed causes less pressure on the perineum. It is more squishy, more stretchy and there is no forced pushing because, the vaginal walls are prepared oxygenated and ready to stretch. This means there is a reduced risk to tear because you are working with your body. And the relaxation of your muscles and focus on the dilation of the cervix and vaginal muscles will also reduce the pressure and requirement for episiotomy.

To slow down pushing even when your body wants to and the contractions are very very strong, you can pant and breathe very slowly exhaling as if you would only cause a candle to flicker if you were blowing into it. Controlled breathing.

So very gently, so very very gently. Breathe out the excess energy of push and breath in the energy of calm breathe out the energy of push and breathe in the energy of flow breathe forward the energy of flow and gently push, so the energy exertion is distributed through the control of the breath and your muscular pushing to reduce pressure on the vaginal walls and perineum.

Here are three intentions - you can make an image of the word push and flow and calm.

Give them a colour to make this very simple.

1. Breathe out any excess, breathe out the colour of "push" and breath in the colour of calm

2.Breathe out the colour of push and breathe in the colour of flow.

3. Breathe forward the colour of flow and gently push with a candle flicker breath. A breath so light that if you were blowing onto a candle, it would stay alight.

This is the same gentility you will use with the self-stimulation. So you can make the pleasure sense build in the moments of comfort between contracts. Very gently, as you pace your own experience.

If you think about it mentally at first it might feel like patting your head and rubbing your tummy at the same time. But in action it's a very synergistic movement, not just physical but movement a primal maternal draw to move with whatever easer pain. A movement of your focus fixation onto breath, pleasure self-pleasure and movement to all encourage comfort and the sensation of pleasure and comfort replacing the prospect of discomfort and pain.

Your breath centres your energy and attention, and as you do you continue or introduce self-pleasure as an additional movement. While repeating some of the below affirmations, my cervix is opening like a flower envisage the diagram, each opening in concentric circles as in dilation as I move towards the birth if my baby.
My body is working with me to birth my baby with ease.
With each contraction I feel a deeper sense of pleasure and can climax easily as a when is most comfortable. My body is working with me to birth my baby with pleasure and ease.

The body can birth a baby into the environment without a controlling mind. [i] So the interception of the thoughts that would interfere with the birth being calm natural and your body birthing baby with ease is achieved as you work through this book and especially "Powerful positivity for childbirth. "
If we elude the thoughts that would prelude an uncomfortable birth.
By way of hypnosis and relaxation with guided suggestion to the contrary then a comfortable birth should prevail. So actively focusing your consciousness on supportive mechanisms and visualisations will clear the way for a more comfortable birth. Visualising creating sensations of calm and visualising the sensations of opening of the cervix in colour in your mind's eye...are just two examples of how your mind can focus to actively support you birthing baby.

Your cervix...
The circles each relaxing, concentric circles.
Opening like a flower with each breath of relaxation you experience.

To red to orange to yellow too green and to blue. Expanding at your bodies chosen pace. As you centre your attention on the wave of each contraction concentric circles opening at your bodies chosen pace. "

If you choose you can colour the circles by hand in this book. Own them and embed the words above. The episiotomy is not essential nor the pushing or size of the baby nor any singular cause for the need. It is possible that the simple handling of the final stages by controlling your breath, push, and body. Like reversing a large car into a small space – add in a multi-storey car park so your perception is enclosed, and you have the idea. It's a precision, you can adhere and achieve through the control of your body and breathing through relaxation fixation, and arousal and positioning alone. But it takes practice.

Stage two labour and birth

The contractions will strengthen but last only around 45 seconds to one minute. Then you have 2 – 5 minutes rest even at their peak.

Your cervix will be fully dilated, you will feel pressure great pressure in your vagina and in your abdomen. Pushing ensues and you will move with the rhythm of your body as your body needs to push and it's safe to push you push. Your clitoris is a central place for pleasure and its surrounding areas as you massage them and breathe.

You can feel a sense of arousal when you are breathing so you remain calm confident and in control. You are breathing baby down bearing down.

As you breathe baby breathes.

Pushing lasts for up to 3 hours maximum. But is likely to be more efficient.

At the birth, as baby crowns should your position be optimum you may experience a g spot activation internally as baby crowns, these moments are so fast and in your mind will feel like a heartbeat.

When baby is born you will deliver the placenta, potential for intervention is always present such as forceps venteuse, caesarean, even if you have a textbook delivery and perform all things well, then, the placenta may require manual removal, there are many things which could happen. That cannot be accounted for however, should they happen, you can remain calm, confident and in control. And always perceive of everything you have done and endured as an accomplishment. Because you birthed, and that's not a nothing. It's a very important something.

" AFFIRMATIVE... CAPTAIN "

" ... WHAT YOUR MIND CONCEIVES YOUR BODY CAN ACHIEVE "

Positive affirmations for child birth

My babies birth will be incredible.
An experience shared with my partner.
Any fears belong to another space another place another time and irrelevant to the birth of this baby
My body was designed and built to birth this baby with ease.
I am relaxed and I am happy that my baby is about to be born. Each contraction has a job to do – Once this con-

traction is complete I will never experience this contraction again.

I am looking forward to each contraction

I am working in partnership with my baby

As I am calm my baby will be so.

As I am relaxed my body will birth my baby efficiently My muscles work together by making birth easier.

I relax as we move through each phase of birth as we work at my bodies own pace.

My body is working at its own pace.

My body is positioned perfectly for each stage of labour I will make decisions that are right for me and my baby.

I am in tune with my body.

I am in listening to the messages it keeps sending me I will make decisions that are right for me and my baby I am in tune with my body I am working with the support I have around me.

I am supported within and around me.

I stay centred inside in my world as the world moves around me to birth my baby with ease As change occurs within and around me I stay centred in the eye of the change I am strong, stable and always provided for. After the birth of my baby My vessels contract and my placenta comes away easily after birthing my baby I recover quickly and easily What my mind conceives my body can achieve

As you appreciate now baby is here. You did it. Now the next chapter of your journey begins. Breathing into your life as a mother or a father or a parent. As it sleeps the gentle rise and fall of babies chest as it breathes its first breaths independent of the womb and umbilical cord. I feel a sense of wonder and awe as I appreciate the miracle that is me and My newborn baby You can become absorbed in the miracles of life and enjoy the moments in time fully present in adoration of baby and the your union with it. You birth together. As you do your body will have comfort. You can use everything you have learned to reduce the discomfort. Turn down the sensations of discomfort or pain or strain by using the dials. Move slowly and frequently to ease the discomfort and move into healing.

**MANTRA **I am capable of birthing my baby with ease and confidence. I am a strong and confident woman. I am able, I am loved, I am supported by Life (the universe or your equivalent) within and around me. I am respected, appreciated, honoured. I am enough. I can support my baby fully.

I am strong and always have and am enough to provide for me and my loved ones. I am balanced. I am centred. I am fulfilled each day in meaningful ways as a mother and a woman. I am confident of my ability to birth baby and be a extraordinary parent.

" IT'S ALL ABOUT POSITIONING BABY …. "

*" She dances to the rhythm of her own heartbeat,
and the sounds of her soul " Michelle Schaper*

Positioning and movement to manifest efficiency in labour. Bring harmony, release pressure and to harness the pressure for its natural flow to birth baby more comfortably and more efficiently.

Practicing positioning through all stages of pregnancy will help and give you greater strength and flexibility in your whole body. Also becoming familiar with your body and building a sense of familiarity with pleasuring in different positions. Stretching, and building strengths when you are.

The more you use the positions the easier they will become when you need them, and imagining the first time you use them is when you are 40 weeks pregnant in transitional labour, they will likely be incredibly alien, and ineffectual. It would feel like doing twister the game when youre 40 week pregnant.

Not funny or easy. Each day consistently spend time doing the exercises. building the muscles and strengths i the right places the postures as you go become embedded as natural as you move towards your birthing day

 Though then you use them as you are moving through this book make time. Make space for you each day to prepare for birthing baby.

Much the same as increasing your state of arousal and regular climax through labour. To move your body gives the energy of constriction and tension a means of expulsion so you can turn the tension into calm, using the meditations in the book and repeated affirmations …

My vagina is relaxing to make way for the birth of my baby.

The muscles in my vagina are now relaxing and opening like a flower to give the optimal opening for my baby to enter this world.

I am calm confident and in control.

As I breathe baby breathes

I am calm baby is calm.

My cervix is opening like a flower, a beautiful flower.
My vaginal walls are expanding in relaxation to allow the flow of baby into this world. combined with movement tin stage two labour this will influence your body's ability to birth baby with ease and facilitate faster healing after birth.
Positions to progress efficiency and comfort. All of which are complemented by self play and allow for the progression of orgasm. They complement it in fact and will enhance the ability of your body to experience the sensation of orgasm anatomically.

1. Hands and Knees:

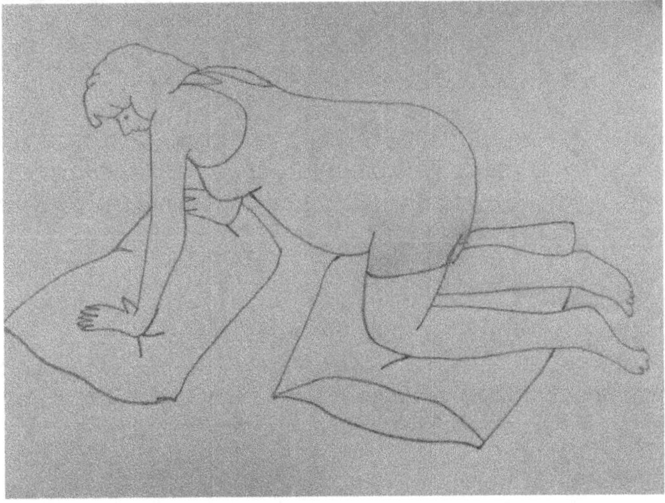

Reduces pressure on the back – spine and allows to stretch the neck back and shoulders.

Reduces pressure on the baby.

Ensure knees and hands supported by pillows and someone

close to offer support a sideways roll.

2.Leap Frog :

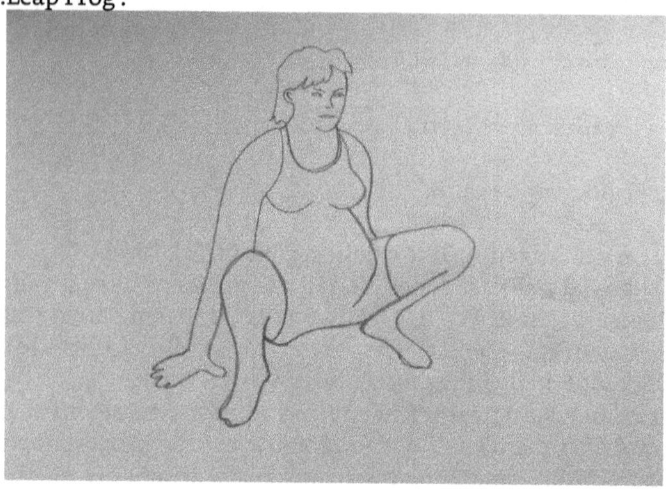

Effects: opening of the pelvic region.

Reduced hip pain by stretching through.

Gives expansion to the shoulders and the back.

Relieves the constriction through stretching and requiring the energy of the body expand into the spaces of movement where it will be naturally Called to the places of the constriction or discomfort.

Moves labour forward through is an effective redirection of your energy into calm movement and flow.

Practice strengthen you knees and ability to resume a stand when using this position while pregnancy progresses.

3. Supported squat:

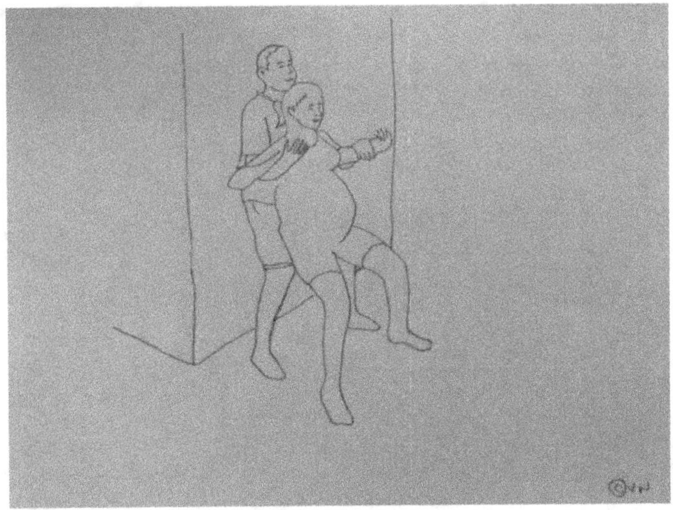

For obvious reasons logistically - supported squat is helpful. Predominantly Gravity.

Benefits: the skin-to-skin contact from the supporter reduces anxiety and stress hormones creating comfort. Reduces anxiety and brings harmony to the body.

Increases oxytocin production.

Stretches the posterior, stretches discomfort through the back and also opening the pelvis and increasingly expelling tension turning it in to comfort. Bringing harmony to the body and mind.

Bouncing in this position may also be helpful.

Pushing your back and pelvis down to release tension until you are ready to push baby through the canal.

4. Any of the following.

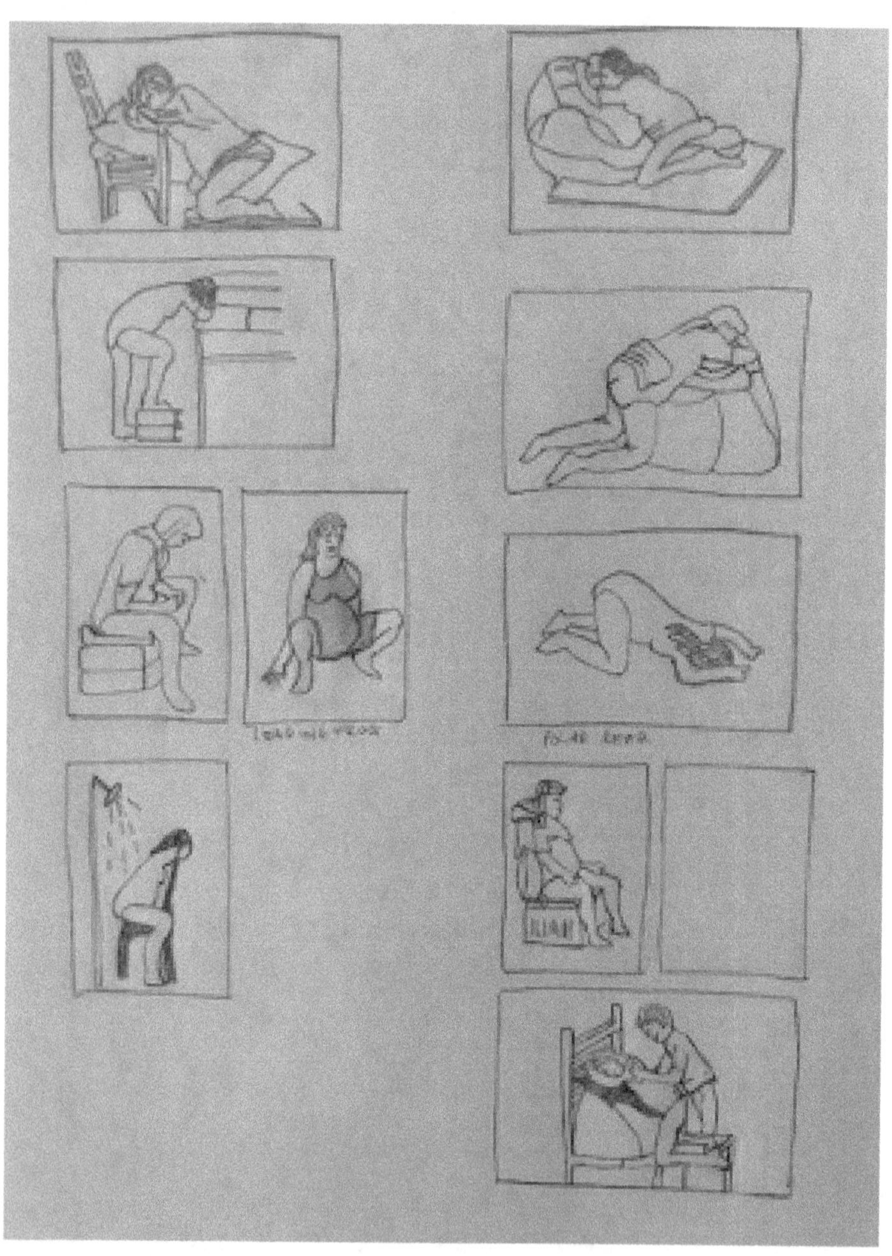

Each position also complements, The Big O principles of accessing the female centres for arousal, and other close bonds with your partner.

The proximity of the spacing between you and your partner

means you are one within union.
The erogenous zones, The vagina, the clitoris, positions for sexual excitement, and the coalescence of the seats of arousal within positioning.

As you move through contractions, move through waves of contraction on bringing comfort and excitement bringing a sense of union with your body baby and partner. The sense of intimacy and love that becomes you as a central focus in labour. The synergy of body working with you and you working with your body to birth baby with ease.

This occurs in any birth, with the integration of the orgasmic template you become more fluid, where there is less medication you are more lucid yet also entranced by the experience itself. You are more aware, and your experience in this way is very primal, but with a bond of love and absolute support that is so very palpable and real. That you have everything you need to manage you level of pain but also to bring a harmony to your birth experience which is unprecedented. To experience the confidence to work with your body as you have learned to engage with the orgasmic template and overlay it at exactly the points where you need it the most.
Knowing your body you will know when these times are and you will know how to move at a pace that is exactly right for you. Everything covered in this book builds and seals and works together layer by layer. So when you finally need it in the moment of birthing it will be there already integrated. Loaded prepared for your experience.
A harmony to your experience which is beyond your expectation.

Now you know, The cycle of arousal, What an orgasm is the stages how to make them, how to harness them, The female sexual body, now you know, and can identify, what an orgasm is. The stages of orgasm. The layers and how they can translate into the stages of child birth and it actually makes sense when it is overlayed

Thy types of orgasm, an introduction to your body, and the places you can make excite to make that happen and how to make them happen.

Your uterus. Its intricate structure. The emerging purpose of the orgasmic template.

The stages of labour and what it means to overlay the orgasmic template, through your birthing experience. The chemical sequences, how to orchestrate the synergy of your dynamic organic structures and sequences, and how it makes sense so you can use it. You are familiar with your uterus, it's role function and form and your erogenous zones, places to try places to learn and places to love.

You know the intricate structure of your uterus, the pain pleasure paradigm, how to reverse pain sensations, how to breathe to pervade calm, the mind body connection, the purity of the origination of your physical makeup on. A cellular level and how to influence this with each act thought word and deed. The construction, production and mixture of biochemical synergy that occurs in labour and orgasm, the orgasmic template overlaying birth.

The process and progress of labour, what will happen how it will feel and what to do when it does, you know how to control your energy and focus when birthing, how to move your body and position for ease. To overlay the orgasmic template in labour step by step at your very own pace. When and how to move your body in synergy with the flow of labour, for efficiency and comfort.

CHAPTER SIX

" There is nothing more rare or more beautiful than a woman being unapologetically herself comfortable in her imperfect imperfection. To me that is the true essence of beauty "

" But the result of all the telling only deepens the enigma and makes women's erotic force something that male storytelling can never explain or contain "

Accepting Female sensuality in birth - Overcoming Social and ecological challenges to Birthing babies with the Big O.

These concepts are a very much hypothetical to sample and soften the the inner rejections to the possibility that this could work for you, and that you are strong enough, sensitive enough to allow it to be so.

Religion, culture are very very strong loyalties in life, but the belief that all can be honoured while still exercising the right to birth a baby with less pain and perhaps so analgesia as a possibility and potential reality.

The aim to see the good in all facets and pursue a path that brings your birth most comfort. With respect for the grace of god, your divinity and your ability to make up your own mind also.

A woman who births is a powerful force in this world and as such the aspect of her body and mind in acceptance that she can birth in her chosen way is to be accepted as the norm. Just as previously and in some place's hospitalisation, epidurals are the norm there will be a time in the future when birthing babies by overlaying the orgasmic template to facilitate birth will be as commonplace as hypnobirthing is now. The transitional shift will come through education, through a change in the direction of beliefs formed over of conflict with social etiquette and religious practice. Harmony can be brought though all with education and a fixation upon the science and the actuality of the construct presented.

Your body is capable of so much more than we had previously perceived so the exploration and acceptance of the potential

can now bring honour to the act of orgasmic birth. Honour to you as a woman and honour to you as a birthing mother.
This is a huge leap in the consciousness of what is acceptable for your birthing experience but the potential is also huge.

There will be a natural disparity in the idealisation of climactic birth however, it's different.

When a woman can bring about a birth, even eliminating discomfort calling her body in union by act to work with her to birth her baby with less pain more efficiently. Completely independently.

Acceptance of female sexuality overcoming embarrassment and the re-establishment of acceptance of the female sexual expression requires education and appreciation.

There is an immense condescendence of the unity on the woman in her strength and assertion of power, which does not always present itself as an overt judgement. But as a undercurrent in any particular flow of their lives at some place it will be present, and can be healed. It can be healed.

This is not to say that orgasmic birth should be the topic of conversation at your birth announcement gender reveal or even Christmas dinner, what's to say if you really accept it as a possibility and a right course of action for you, within you. You may not even ever need to defend it. You own it and therefore it is you. Its your choice. Make sure you own the construct before you share it.

The leap is to formulate a firm distinction between carnal desire and the intention to overlay the orgasmic template in childbirth.

It's a high probability that once you introduce the orgasmic template as a concept, questions, fears, and preconceptions arise within. There will be judgements, conversations, curiosities, even sniggers, it's natural.

This said, the perception and overshadowing is vast in to say that the woman is not enough to sustain or maintain the of birth but to carry the child to birth the baby feed and nourish the baby is already within her. As is her ability to birth the baby independently. She does not have to, but she can as if she chooses to.

The recognition of her ability to birth and also as such her ability to call in the assistance of others to facilitate the birth of baby neither of which demean or weaken her because she is strong, and able as a birthing mother.

The illusion of alternate truths from others perceptions over-laid to now can be any means, maybe family members of parentage,religious commitments the ignorance and condescendence that exists as an undercurrent surrounding female sexual familiarity. Or where pleasure in a woman of a carnal nature is prohibited in religion, even law in some countries.

Primarily the preconceptions which come with sexual explorational familiarity. Promiscuity versus education and experience.

Often viewed that women's who are sexually familiar and experienced are somehow lower or worthless, that they are experienced because they are promiscuous or that they are cheapened by their expression of desires and exploration for sexual preferences.

Shame of sexual expression relative to promiscuity, or as a symptom of the repulsion of purity in the interaction relative to experience. That someone must have been so active as to be so experienced in knowledge when in truth many of the aspects they have graduated into in their experience could have come from a book and a direct adherence to the mastery of a skill, while still respecting the purity of their own belief or imposition of what is right for them.

To enhance quality without increasing quantity in the pursuit of knowledge and experience in other ways.

Women and men face a conundrum of mixed messages about sex while living in a culture that exploits sex and women on the one hand and makes judgement freedom of expression on the other.

The variants tend to be around promiscuity and the perception of the degree of experience directly relative to having met with more people. The degree of experience being linked with multiples of partners.

The two are only linked by perception therefore can be un-founded as long as a woman and man are of sexual health then should be no judgement as to whether someone has more or less sexual partners. Experience can be gained from a book and elegantly interwoven so does not necessarily pur-port to a higher number of sexual partners.

Studies show that women tend to underestimate the num-ber of sexual partners they have had during their lifetime; whereas men are more likely to exaggerate them. Perhaps as a loyalty and cleanliness binding the feminine to her purity being dependent on innocence in an archaic form on some archetypical level. However, aside sexual health this should not be a vital concern. From others to the woman but moder-ated by the woman in her own mind as to what is right and wrong and acceptable for her within her own new expanded parameters.

Researchers from Cornell University found that among 500 women surveyed, a hypothetical woman who had more than 20 partners was considered "less competent and emotionally stable, less warm, and more dominant" than a hypothetical woman who had only two sexual partners. These findings resonate with the belief that women ought to be modest and suppress, or, worse, feel ashamed of their sexual interest and longing. A relational fall-out from this double standard is that it incentivizes people to conceal the truth about sexual past experiences. But guilt and dishonesty are deadly issues in a relationship. Because it leads to incumbency and subordin-ation. Perhaps because of the repeated sense of loss on a pri-mal scale of the building of familiarity and then of the partner being withdrawn. When we are programmed to have on one level one mate for life.

In building the confidence of a woman, to turn the confidence within and suggest that the unity they have within, to the aspects of themselves that are the male and the female, the respect and unity which they would perceive as another is within them of their own, so they are loyal to the self who is in fact them so they are their mate for life. They can choose to reflect it to another to make bonds and much the same can re-tain the trajectory of their own. This is a deep construct. But let it percolate, it's purely on an archetypical level. They are forgiving of past encounters accepting of their strength and develop the warmth towards self and others because the space of the union is within themselves. Welcoming the union and therefore pure, within the parameters of their acceptance. They are experienced because they enjoy making love, they enjoy their body and the experience of the sensation in their body.

In birthing babies possibly the only dominant reason which pervades the interaction between sexual experience and pleasure in birth is the science. This is a scientific, empirically evidenced course of action which can lead to a birthing with less pain, to enhancing the bond you have with your body with your baby with your birth and even with your partner.

For a woman to embrace her self respect and acceptance, and realise that she has within her " self ".

The Place of worship the Trust.

Love acceptance.

Freedom to make choices.

Acceptance of her femininity.

Acceptance of the male.

The sense of safety in the space of union.

Passion, Intimacy, commitment will ensue, concurrent with her ability to climax in her chosen way and experience whichever climatic experiences she chooses. This is the foundation of the improvement of quality and experience of sexual interactions. They needn't be great in number or frequency though can be of extreme quality.

It's important to make the distinction between carnal desire and the urgency, the primal urgency to make movements towards reducing the sensation of pain in birth. Your motive in calm is centered, and to experience pleasure to alleviate pain.

Being experienced and familiarity with your body is an advantageous position, to be encouraged. When you are educated, because it relates less to experimentation with multiple partners but in fact gives you guidance and confidence to explore your own body. Its your body and you can explore it without shame. To build confidence in this exploration and to appreciate it. The religious, and condescendence of social perceptions of sexual pleasure and feminine empowerment are very misplaced in this context.

The researchers also surveyed men with identical information about a male peer—20 partners versus two. The subjects rated the more sexually active male as "more competent and emotionally stable" than the hypothetical male who had two sexual partners.

These are just perceptions, overwhelmingly.

Can you watch porn to mimic the sensations. Yes possibly, advised in context no.

The intention within is the difference, if a woman asserts self pleasure to birth baby with fixation in her mind of pain relief. That is a very different position to stand in than watching pornographic content for joy. There is no reason why two people cannot watch porn together and then embrace their own sexual desires in alignment with that if that is their choice and will is the external perception which causes the disparity and the extent that the external perception may dominate the internal perception and sense of what is right and wrong.

In Many cultures it is a different, defensible in a very different vein. Is porn an effective place to search to for education about sexual conduct ... NO.

Self exploration is. Pornographic content has it's place, but not for education.

If that is your chosen way. Yes great.

As long as that is embraced and acknowledge true acceptance of pleasure can ensue. Without the shame.

In the modern age female sexuality is begging to be accepted more in its expression and freedom through there are so many taboos about leadership and the expression and fulfilment of feminine sexual desires. Firstly giving permission within experience sexual pleasure.

The idea of feminine sexual expression in some belief structures and cultures is so far from the perception within western cultures. It is hidden undisclosed and undiscussed. Shamed and frowned upon. The era when it is acceptable for women to be open about their sexuality is upon us. Woman are opening about their sexual freedom and they can begin to experience the freedom of self-expression without the stigma attached.

There are cultural barriers, religious barriers all of which begin to permeate the strength of a woman to express herself sexually but these barriers, are beginning to be moved through and beyond. Sexual freedom and expression, to experience the greatest sexual pleasures and to do in a way in harmony with her femininity especially when pregnant and labouring is a step beyond the traditional parameters of actualisation. The barriers include Religion, predominantly and religion is good, belief is good strong moral ethos is good, Faith is good. It's how the faith is held within you that sometimes purports to a challenge that's is overcome- able. Looking at each on in turn, allows a perspective shift so valuable that cannot not see the value in the possibility to expand your sexual freedoms in a way that compliments all areas of your beliefs and that it is possible to do so without fear judgement or prejudice. Once you see the window for that possibility then you can .

The main cultural barriers so sexuality are far reaching, in Asia a lack of sexual desire is reported to be held to be normal as women are " not allowed " to have sexual desires. And the dictated dedication to a god, maintaining the family honour and perpetuation of the preconception of purity being associated with diminished desire or freedom to express. To be pure on has no desires of a sexual nature. With the consequences for deviation being great. To grasp the sentiment that you can have sexual desires and be pure in the light of god is a leap for many. The privacy of the space of the woman to respect her religion is vital. In all cultures this may not be an applicable practice though that does not reflect on it is effectiveness simply whether it is a good fit.

Catholicism places women at the role of subservience, sexual morality strict honour codes and passivity the care giving role and self-sacrifice with the condemnation of the pleasure and purpose of creation to be the only advancement of sexual enticement for as to grow the colony of the servitor. More expansion to the devout beliefs means that it is possible to honour religious beliefs and to experience great sexual pleasure. This simply means allowing oneself to experience the joys of the feminine pleasure. Accepting that pleasure is not a sin and that in fact is a form of union with spirit, a celebration of God and all that is pure. In the union of the desires of a woman and man in intimacy. To overcome the perpetration that a woman cannot feel pleasure because it is not permitted or supported by their belief in servitude to God, is to ensure they are supported by their own god within. However the represent this to themselves.

Masculine presence as macho and dominant, overbearing and these are strong stereotypes to overcome and work through. Male dominance and power are strong connections especially in India and eastern world where women are placed as sub lower and more inferior where-as the scope of a woman's strength is through matriarchal line. The accumulation of their essences as a matriarch combined in comparison to man in a different perspective these can support the notion for sexual pleasure as an advancement of childbirth in turn to bring comfort. And to enshrine the union of the matriarch the mother and the lover into one who can choose to experience great pleasure.

The thing is to balance the concept of gods will.

In many cultures childbirth is to be endured without expectation or the offer of comfort. In indigenous cultures women birth alone without relief, in contrast to the lack of distraction suggestion and the media preconceptions of intervention and hospitalisation being a norm. Women are expected to birth naturally and do so more often without complication. In private, in a sacred space, where no or very little medical facility is available.

Quite often you will find that it's the concept of sexual pleasure and acts of sexual nature which prelude to something shameful or even embarrasing. This is not so because like with all act's actions it's the intention behind the act which influences the act itself. That given in this context to birth baby with comfort. To use something so natural such as the orgasmic template. To make babies entry to the word as healthy and chemically free experience or to ensure that you once again claim your mental perspective and once again prelude the purity of the act of arousal as pleasure is pure. To some cultures this ideal is so far from grace that it would be banished. Though. It remains.

When sexual satisfaction is said to be something which

causes disparity in the relationship for the feminine, that it blurs the relationship with God. It isn't, that god does not will the pleasure to the woman in her mind. It's the forgiveness of the woman to herself for finding the god within such that she can permit herself to experience the pleasure. In consideration of her motive. the distinguishing principle in the definition of the act and the direction of the attention energy and transmutation is what is your motive.

When you are ain acceptance of your motive then
 To accept that is is ok.

The bible and books of all religion can be inverted, subverted and interpreted in any way to prove any man or woman's principles correct. The point is to be the one who chooses to make her own perception even with the devout service to God. That does not hinder a woman's ability or opportunity to experience fulfilment if she so chooses, nor does it hinder her ability to make peace with that in her own mind. The acceptance of the woman to know she is loved and supported by her god who would grant her pleasure as along as she in the honour of her own code of belief. Especially when she is overlaying the orgasmic template within childbirth. To bring the experience of pain to a minimum and to encourage a woman in her physical body defined by god to use it in its greatest capacity to fulfil the role it was designed to fulfil. Birth baby. To relate to god, the woman was born with a clitoris for the purpose of pure pleasure, to be so intricately made with the inclusion of this then it must be gods will that the woman can use her body to define her own parameters of pain. Especially in the act of child birth.

To expand the belief such that she can be fulfilled as much as the man in ways she chooses. So that she can serve, but also to serve herself of the pleasures which she envisions of the others. Such as granting the male the freedom of her body so to can she grant herself the permission to experience and exercise this freedom and privilege herself too.

Within the motive of childbirth.

It takes a leap for you to internally justify the approach, however, you do that that is Ok. As long as you are fully welcoming and committed to making this work for you it will.

Once you give yourself permission to do this. Permission is a powerful force, to bring paths into union and to make forward a very potent solution. Always centred, and aware of your motive.

In building confidence to overlay the template in practice, when imagining self pleasure within child birth, it will appear different when you are in the moment every aspect you have read in this book will make sense and the sensation will be very different than the perception of past experience of carnal desire and love. This said there are key parallels, between comfort and familiarity in the birthing environment to reduce the sense of stressors. Relatively in terms of female expression key elements must be present.

Sternberg [32]

Includes three major components:
(1) passion,
(2) intimacy,
(3) commitment.

These are all huge pre cursers underpinning the sense of safety which will prelude intimacy and expression and a sense of self-acceptance which is more likely to occur when all these three are present.

They are relative to birthing as such.

(1) Focus fixation intention (

2) Appreciation of the body – Tuning into the sensations in the body

(3) The sense of familiarity – Safety.

That they are secure with their partner or secure within themselves and secure within their mind and body as to the expression of their own personal desires and preferences. The depth of the arousal available to the woman and man is dependent on these contingents. That they are safe and feel so, that they are secure and they feel so.

In birthing when women are secure in their environment their nervous system will reflect this. Birth will progress more purposefully, and the instinctive stressors, which are often unidentifiable. Are reduced. So the body can relax in to the experience of birth or the experience of intimacy to it s fullest most harmonious extent.

Their body and their own Sexual motives. Acceptance will naturally vary from culture to culture. In most cultures sexuality is viewed as an expression of love, devotion, and intimacy, of finesse and grace. Which is how you can carry the motive forward in birthing.

In truth the key components to overcome the stigma and perpetuation of the overbearing religious context. Not necessarily as a cause to fight within society but within ones own mind. This is the only place resolution can be found into acceptance. The resolution of ones own thinking on what is acceptable within the parameters of thier own beliefs the structure of their life their family and everywhere in between. To balance this with your new found parameter of belief and to find a space for your own acceptance and ownership of what it is that you are choosing and enjoying in the induction of this change. By way of your good motive to birth your baby with great comfort.

Where women are so strongly held in the space of being fearful of the gods or the perpetration of the power of a god in dominance.

Your god knows your motive is good, and therefore supports your path.
Is more effectual this way. More over that they can experience the pleasure within safe haven should they be required to do so.

They can experience the pleasure knowing they have a deeper connection with the faith in themselves that that they deserve to experience pleasure and to experience the depth of satisfaction comfort and love.
That what will come about is the love within the union of the self in mind.
It's to give herself permission to express her choices desires

and pleasure. Within the realm of acceptance by herself and that of her partner.

To have faith that her self-love is as powerful as the love she has for her religious beliefs that the two beliefs and structures will complement each other and respect each other so she can indeed move forward and take great strength in the space of being loved accepted as a person within their own right to make choices to honour her religion in any way of her choosing. This is bold but it is also quiet and, and quiet as a whisper of her soul in her space that makes her feel so much more secure.

When she feels secure, and all her belief structures are complementary the things she holds greatest to her religion and her honour.

All of the below are essential essences in intimacy.
And are mirrored in birth.

Honour for her space of worship.

Trust

Love

Acceptance

Freedom to make choices.

Acceptance of her femininity

Acceptance of the male and the sense of safety in the space of union.

Passion intimacy and commitment will ensue.

When she feels comfortable orgasmic pleasure is greater and more heightened and the sense pleasure is experiences through her whole being and sense of self.

To even begin to imagine the context of sexual desire and pleasure and for purpose is an alien concept to many women who are enshrined within the vows under the religious or cultural beliefs, but this can change. And is beginning to evolve as western society begins to accept the place of sexual exploration.

Pleasure oneself to be accepted and to be enjoyed, is the movement forward, to express sexual desires openly with a partner or in the birthing suite and to be accepting of the space of her own mind and body to actualise these desires and expressions is becoming more accepted.

Female expression of sexual desires and dominance. The expression of a woman and her ability to make choices to pleasure herself. To dominate and to assert. To instigate. More acceptable without the tarnishing of her character or the assumption of promiscuity to be linked or connected with that of pleasure and experience. Quality is not necessarily related to quantity. Expression to build a solid sexual experiential and experimental repertoire does not mean with multiple people in necessity so has no connection in connotation but to build the confidence of a woman to freely express herself means an adornment of security and an advancement of confidence that is the beginning of expression. And grows through time. Because it is one with her motive.

A deep and real connection to the self and an allowance of the ability to fee real pleasure and feel the pleasure of sexual expression and indulgence is a birth right to all women, whatever has preceded them or been learned by them. It means they have the ability and opportunity within them heal it, to experience this opening and to enjoy that. To forgive what has been, and love into what could be, and enjoy a new time.

To have faith that herself love is as powerful as the love she has for her religious beliefs that the two beliefs and structures will complement each other, and respect each other. She can indeed move forward and take great strength in the space of being loved, accepted as a person within their own right to make choices to honour her religion in a way of her choosing. This is bold but it is also quiet and, and quiet as a whisper of her soul in her space that makes her feel so much more secure.

When she feels secure, and all her belief structures are complementary the things she holds greatest to her religion and her honour. She is stronger and more aligned more certain and more confident. In her chices and acts. Passion intimacy and commitment will ensue herby enhancing the depth of the intensity of the auric presence of the feminine of the soul in her strength and most beautiful as a flame of desire.

In developed countries such developed countries continue to strive for equality for women and men regardless of orientation, race, or ethnicity. Gender equality requires fair treatment, positive regard, respect, and acceptance of difference. Partnership equality relies on the integration that all parts fit together to create a collective whole, striving toward wholeness through cooperation, responsibility, and contribution.

Though women often seem to be at risk of discrimination and subversion this can and is changing every day in small ways. Some greater power is born to the woman even in ways unnoticeable until they build momentum. In life consistency builds momentum and in life momentum wins.

Women have achieved definite success toward not subjugating their needs to their male counterparts. Union and teamwork mean Working together, where one has weakness the other grows to support, as opposed to rising to subordinate the weaker, they will raise to fill the void to bolster. So, she is not weak she is loved. And the same on the alternate side. You rise to fill the void and then the union merges and bends as is needed that is the notion of relationship of the whole of the partnership, they are synergistic. Coalescent. The ebb and flow of the power and strength moves between them they can both be strong and then they can both be weak though the union usually flows as such that the essence of the union is of ebb and flow where the shift in strength of the masculine and the feminine and the relative qualities of each, are shared that is the nature of marriage. That is the nature of the essence of a matrimonial partnership even if you are not "married in law".

So, for the purposes of overcoming cultural and social dynamics pervading a woman's ability to embrace her sexuality and increase her confidence towards the inclusion of arousal and orgasm in her birthing journey. The fixation of the intention within the arousal is of the birthing journey, It is different as mentioned earlier, when this is the intention. But in order for the woman to experience arousal she must be permitted to by herself, to accept it and even privately enjoy the experience.

To engage and embody birth, and embody the sensation of arousal so as to progress birth with the strongest intention to feel less pain. The distinction between carnal desire and primal incentive to reduce discomfort is very clear.

Evidence shows pleasurable birth experiences are characterised by sexual, physical sensations with no accompanying erotic ideation in regard to the foetus, and yet the concept still evokes stigmatisation.

Anonymous online forums such as Mumsnet.com show these women to be depicted as 'perverted' (Caffrey, 2014).

The shame associated with sexual birth experiences is particularly evident within the UK study, where women would use terms such as 'sensual' and 'pleasurable' without acknowledging the sexual dimensions of these sensations (Caffrey, 2014). Harel's study (2007) additionally showed that with three of the interviewees, there was admission of feeling the need to 'hold back' sexually. This discomfort was a result of the presence of others at the birth, shame and lack of privacy (Harel, 2007). Accept that sexual arousal in this context outside of the bedroom is acceptable.

Yet when you have the perception that this is science. This isn't perverted even if it is erotic to the core because that is what is intended it's one of the purest forms of pain relief. However, for some people to grasp that is a great leap especially generationally and culturally. The general theme is if you are ok with it, that's great. But it's something that I would suggest you speak about sensitively with trusted companions. Because some people just won't get it and that is to be expected. And accepted. Though you will get it. You are reading this, so do get it.

You have the science. You have also the reminder that you don't need everyones approval all of the time to be able to progress with a concept. You embrace it and make it your own. Or to approve of yourself, your choices. And make it work as your own. Despite this, at present, the only reference made to a woman's sexual wellbeing in her pregnancy within antenatal guidelines surround the safety of sexual intercourse, enquiring about sexual trauma, and undertaking clinical tests for sexually transmitted infections (NICE, 2008).

Sex within midwifery practice therefore remains clinical and disconnected from the woman's identity, omitting the concept of pleasure and passion within birth. In addition to the lack of formal midwifery education regarding the connections between sexuality and birth experience, the practitioner's own lack of confidence or views regarding discussing sexuality may prevent effective communication (Foux, 2008; Nelson, 2009). So be strong enough to approach the topic with your midwife, you can initiate a dignified and inclusive conversation, and you may be pleasantly surprised by their response.

Be open and communicate, be strong enough in your education and commitment to gently assert a your choice, and explain. As you would do if you were using hypnotic birthing practices.

Evidence also suggests the potential of antenatal education for prospective parents. When reviewing both studies by Harel (2007) and Caffrey (2014), the education of the women interviewed appeared to influence their openness to engage with their sexuality within the intrapartum period. Women reported that the inclusion of childbirth as a positive, physiological, and potentially ecstatic event within antenatal education was, or would have been, beneficial in supporting their experiences (Caffrey, 2014). Most of the women recognised that sexuality and pleasure were part of birth, and actively made attempts to incorporate them, with women claiming the inclusion of intimacy improved the birth progress. The use of nipple or clitoral stimulation as an alternative therapy also warrants further consideration and study, based on the anecdotal reports by women who utilised it as positive, effective pain relief. There are studies which present a clinical significance of the reduction of pain reception before during and before after orgasm when the body is sexually aroused. That is a given and has been studies and evidences by Whipple since the 1970s after experimentation on Rats (which I neither support or condemn personally or professionally in the modern age)

Finally, and most pertinent The role of the birthing environment.

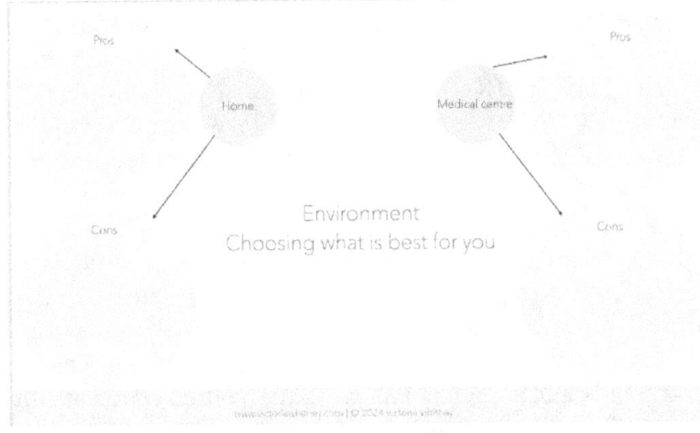

The World Health Organization's (2018) recommendations for a positive birth highlight women's desire for both a clinically and psychologically safe environment during intrapartum care. Intimate settings are essential for women to fully engage in labour, experience calm and exercise the sexual qualities of birth. But with relaxation you can overcome the sense of overwhelm before it even becomes a prospect or ensues. You could contend the environmental disparity between hospital and home.

You can choose, but you are the centre and the commonality within both, so to be calm confident and in control and bring baby into this life calmly in your chosen feel is a conscious choice of you and the energy you are running within your body which is a result of the thoughts you are running in your mind.
So, the preparation for birth begins 9 months before you enter the birthing suite or begin to birth at home. You may choose pain relief, you may not, but your choice is your own and so you own the choice and the act so whatever you choose, feel good about it. Be confident enough to request private spaces, and to assert and use arousal in clinical environments. Welcoming the progression to a time when this is accepted even encouraged, is a current stance.

The choice of birth environment will also determine the analgesia available to women, which in turn may influence the possibility of ecstatic birth. Gaskin (2003) observed that the presence of orgasmic birth is greatly reduced in women whose labours are medicated with narcotics, epidurals, or barbiturates. The options for pharmacological analgesia are limited within a home birth setting in the UK but include inhalational Entonox (a 50:50 mixture of oxygen and nitrous oxide) and opioids (National Institute for Health and Care Excellence [NICE], 2014), with availability dependent on local guidance. Within a hospital environment, women are given the option of epidural analgesia in addition to the above.

Having worked in healthcare for over 20 years I have attended many NHS trainings and the proposition that one day there will be a course or class approved by the midwives that would include this topic. That it would be a normal CPD course much like any of the others, like PSE in school which offers another opportunity to women another pathway.
Whether we can progress to a place where that is acceptable and do so with grace.
To reduce and eliminate the fears brought about by the exploration of your own beliefs bringing your intention, once again to how do you intend your birth, your experience the reception of your family, friends, how much are they included, once you can identify your choices then you can very gently assert them and enjoy the assertion of these choices. As it comes to life.

Now you know, The cycle of arousal. What an orgasm is the stages how to make the, how to harness them, The female sexual body, you can identify What an orgasm is, The stages of orgasm, The layers and how they can translate into the stages of child birth and it actually makes sense when it is overlayed

Thy types of orgasm, an introduction to your body, and the places you can make excite to make that happen and how to make them happen.

Your uterus. It's intricate structure and the emerging purpose of the orgasmic template.

The stages of labour and what it means to overlay the orgasmic template, through your birthing experience. The chemical sequences, how to orchestrate the synergy of your dynamic organic structures and sequences, and how it makes sense so you can use it. You are familiar with your uterus, its role function and form and your erogenous zones, places to try places to learn and places to love.

You know the intricate structure of your uterus, The pain

pleasure paradigm, how to reverse pain sensations, how to breathe to pervade calm, the mind body connection, the purity of the origination of your physical makeup on. A cellular level and how to influence this with each act thought word and deed. The construction, production and mixture of biochemical synergy that occurs in labour and orgasm, the orgasmic template overlaying birth.

The process and progress of labour, what will happen how it will feel and what to do when it does, you know how to control your energy and focus when birthing, how to move your body and position for ease. To overlay the orgasmic template in labour step by step at your very own pace. When and how to move your body in synergy with the flow of labour, for efficiency and comfort.

The divergence of carnal desire and overlaying the orgasmic template in birth. Acceptance of the feminine and your ability to bridge the divide in religious social and cultural beliefs and condescension. How to bridge the cultural and generational divide mentally so you can find acceptance that overlaying the orgasmic template is acceptable. The definition of the space of union in the feminine and encouragement to embrace the contrast in life. The importance and essentials for intimacy and how they are mirrored in birth. And you have the ability to communicate with your midwife, introduce the concept. And hold strong in your personal assertion in choice.

CHAPTER SEVEN

BRINGING IT ALL TOGETHER

" Make the upcoming hour overflow with joy, and let pleasure drown the brim. " William Shakespere.

Rejoice in the possibility of an alternate avenue to generalised pain relief. The expansion of the concept. Though different types of pain. The application of a principle broadened to other forms of pain. As a concept and practice in potential. Applications beyond birth to make your time in reading even more valid over a lifetime.

This theory is applied when exploring the potential of orgasm as an alternative mode of analgesia (Mayberry and Daniel, 2016). Human studies have demonstrated that genital self-stimulation can elevate pain thresholds, activating a powerful analgesic process, that is distinctly separate from a distraction process (Whipple and Komisaruk, 1988; Komisaruk and Whipple, 2000). Studies show that when pleasurable vaginal stimulation is applied, a woman's pain threshold can increase by over 75% and by over 100% in those who experience orgasm, (Whipple and Komisaruk, 1988; Komisaruk and Sansone, 2003).. The Tertiary concept of the cultural beliefs around medicalisation. The culture of hospitalisation. And clinicalisation. The sterility of the hospitalised environment and is not synonymous with sexuality in childbirth (Buckley, 2010; Mayberry and Daniel, 2016). It is suggested that we can already concede that many of the barriers highlighted in many studies about the environment birth occurs in, in fact we often talk about the mind body connection and using arousal to match the natural progression of labour to diminish sensations of pain. The whole premise of Birthing babies with the Big O Is to birth babies with less pain.
To extend this concept to generalised, chronic pain, is a new and interesting concept. And has great potential.

The application in generalised pain relief comes with great caution. It is important to make sure your pain is thoroughly assessed by a medical practitioner. When you have a diagnosis, the source of the pain is diagnosed then this is a suitable option moving forwards but only then. When you have a diagnosis.

Much like in childbirth obviously use of any practices and will be in line with the care of the woman's obstetrics practitioner. So, it's safe and responsible to use climactic pain relief and hypnotherapy for childbirth to reduce the sensation of pain in child birth.
In general terms your pain as a warning get it checked, prior to instigating any pain management routine.

Imagine the possibility of using your mind to experience great relief from chronic pain.
Where pain medication does not work or for those who have an allergy to pain relief. Just the possibilities. It begs you to question what else is our body capable of.

The possibilities are great for the expansion of pain relief through the manipulation of your joy hormones to literally reverse the concept of pain into pleasure.

When the pleasure sensations flood your nervous system the flushes through the pain receptors and with repeated induction with repeated use, like within hypnosis called fractionation each time it becomes more powerful and deeper.
Each time you reach a sensation of hypnotic induction and come out the next time it becomes easier and deeper, because it is familiar. Much like the sensation of orgasm intended for pain relief. You are learning new ways. Each time you practive you form stronger and stronger beliefs. Stronger and stronger lines of new progressed memory of new paths, of arousal directed purely to the source of the physical anatomical pain.

When you move this way in your mind, it becomes something not illusive but something that can be done. Tuned into when you choose, the more you use it for the pure focus of pain relief it becomes familiar, clinical in some respects with precision and so the pleasure flood can be evoked when you choose. With a thought to keep the sensations of pain under your own control.

How would you do this? Remember check your motive.
By visualisation, repeated visualisation. Visualization of
what would lead to the sensation, which is directly for you
they don't have to be pornographic or elicit. Simply by using a
more directed version, which may not even include images of
anatomy aroused but imagining the sensation of arousal to be
sent to the anatomy in pain to be relieved.
Step one arousal physical.. then... repeatedly
To imagine the sensation as a feeling and bring it to a purely
physical level in mind, that you are imaging the sensation of
pleasure build in an area of the body, in your erogenous zones
just by thinking to them, building the pleasure sense or template then taking a snapshot if you like and moving the sensation to the areas where you feel pain.

Then you re assign the need for the physical act of sexual
stimulation or touch by learning the repeated ignition of the
pleasure centre in your mind. To form a distance between
pain relief and direct arousal is one step further but a step
towards the inclusion of a routine pain management system
just by thought. The key in the distance is to make pain relief
accessible anywhere any time.

Just with any induction this is similar because it leads you
into a state of relaxation and then brings your awareness to
the purpose of the induction. Which is to ignite the pleasure
senses in your body by directing your attention t them and
opening them up. You could feel aroused, but when you repeat and fine tune this to the level where you can simply like
an on off switch take five minutes to focus inside switch mentally the pleasure sensors on to the point where you can even
climax, or reach a level which satisfies the requirement to
flood the senses with pleasure so as to override the sensation
of pain, and then allow the sensation of relaxation to remain
such that you can continue with your daily tasks as much as
possible.

It is far less debilitating than the use of powerful drugs with
relatively few side effects and intimacy with your partner can
become a very different experience, also for pleasure but a
very different type of pleasure. There is parallel but also a very
real distinction where there is a clinical like process to the
induction of the sensation of pleasure. It's a mental condi-
tioning to override the previously laid sensations of pain. And
form once again a new synergy with arousal beyond a sexual

act with a partner that you can instigate independently. Which is considerably more convenient.

In childbirth its natural because you are very much associated into the body, your vagina, your cervix and especially the deeply intimate areas such as the G spot and the vaginal canal. Your breasts they are all involved in the process of birthing, but in contrast, for a headache or for example fibromyalgia, there is a very different order to the pain and frequency. So the approach would be adapted such that it was of a more clinical natural and expanded to the possibilities outside of just child birth. The idea that you would take moment to go somewhere private is a huge leap and most likely not acceptable to have to go to somewhere private and engage in masturbation to bring about an orgasm and flood of pleasure to flush the pain. This isn't the aim. The aim is to make orgasms mental. Then make mental a different physical. By re -routing the sensation of release comfort and release to the area of pain. You make a template of the path to arousal and overlay it in your mind to make it accessible anywhere.

To do this is another leap in perspective. To make a clinical approach to orgasm and arousal and their benefits to extend to other areas of pain relief to distance intimacy and to make this a mental process which can be taken anywhere and used anywhere by fixation of attention.

By making the physical sensations an imagining to distance the vagina, the genitals and the intimacy. One become familiar with the sensation, two, Define strong memory links with the sensation, mental lines which carry the association in your ability to increase the sensations of orgasmic high. Track the physical sensations of pleasure. Galvanise this track. And make them accessible by invocation of one word trigger. Resulting in an increase in the pleasure hormones, by simply exciting the lines of association and memory.

The pain relief intention then becomes dissociated from intimacy, simply the neural pathways you make, as if installing another facet of self which retains your sexual expansion, seperate to the associated memories of access arousal states to be ignited purely for the relief of pain and to flush the sensations of pain from your nervous system. You can step in your mind away from intimacy into pleasure and the manipulation of hormones by thinking. If you were a phone, it

would be like installing a pain relief app. It uses similar lines
to tinder, but it does infact have a very different and clinical
purpose.

It's a real use of the power of the mind for real purpose beyond
stigma. Much like the delineation of cannabis in the modern
day for medical clinical therapeutic purposes.

I remember when I was doing my GCSE's one of my English
essays was discursive about "The misuse of drugs act 1971
and the legalisation of cannabis " and other class b drugs. My
favour was neither, but I did the research, and it was a heated
topic at the time some 25 years ago.

Now you can by CBD oil in a supermarket.

It's that acceptable, and as will become the orgasmic template
where you can not necessarily buy it over the counter but you
can learn it through a book or a course and then use it forever.
Imagine the amount people would save on pain meds if they
used this and got really really good at it.

And that's a similar refinement with orgasmic potential can
be refined, to an ignition of the pleasure sensors at will, by
repeated routing of the neural pathways. Generating new
pathways that are directly purposed to open the pleasure sensations release hormones which relax and open, rather than
constrict. So, you can eventually bring it to just one thought
as if you have a button in your mind to enable you to turn on
the pleasure sensation. To flood your neurology with oxytocin, serotonin, dopamine. Or the sensation of the release of
these as a direct feeling. For example, when someone enjoys a
habit but it is bad for them such as drinking, smoking, drugs,
you can engineer their mind to re create the sensation of the
first puff, the first sip or the sensation of a line of cocaine,
simply by pressing two fingers together reinvoke the sensation so they do not do the physical behaviour of doing the
habit they retain the one thing that was helpful for them and
that is the sensation, but they also know they do not link the
sensation with doing the thing any more, they link the sensation with their ability to control their past addiction because
they already have the feeling inside they were looking for by
doing the routine, ritual of the addiction. They have the rush.

Similarly with tooth ache. Sometimes visualisation is a very powerful tool. The imagination of the insertion of the nova-cane injection and memory of the sensation of numbness spreading through the jaw line is enough to overcome the sensation of toothache. In pain. I did this when I was a newly qualified Hypnotherapist. To enliven the memory very potently, is enough.

Visualisations, to the detail of the coolness of the contents of the syringe entering the gum line and then the warmth the growing numbness and sensation of complete relief almost seeing the syringe as the liquid pushed through the comfort grows as does the numbness. And if you needed to top up imagine it again to manage the resolution of the pain.

(Which you can top up at any time.)

Using this method I managed to still work out at the gym daily and maintain good health in between a dental abscess and an extraction.

As with any of these meditations you must always always always consult a dentist, medical doctor to diagnose and treat the cause of the pain precedent to using pain relief methods. It won't cure an abcess for example but will enable you to move through the time and space of healing much more comfortably.
Using the "big O" you are using a different natural approach through meditation.

What if that could be. It can. With repeated focus. Literally forging new paths in your nervous memory, new paths encoded, which could open doors to a whole new way of living. I wouldn't purport it for recreational use. But for the direct use of the reduction in the sensation of pain. For the treatment of chronic pain. More than to just turn off the sensations of pain but to flood the neurology with a sensation of pleasure, to relax, and open rather than constrict. When the body constricts much like in labour, the sensation of pain is so draining a debilitating that the body and mind constrict. It's like a darkness and constriction that pervades the body, mind and soul. When you increase the amount of pleasure hormones day by day the beginning of the relaxation is there, there will through time become less constriction because, you are encoding new paths in the nervous system.
If you imagine a path through a field. The more times some-

one walks this path the more defined the path becomes until it becomes THE accepted and most used path. It requires maintenance and renewal. But the path once forged is there. As before with fractionation the body will not constrict to the same degree. Neuro plasticity is defined – loosely as the intrinsic ability of the nervous system to change adapt and modify its activity in response to intrinsic or extrinsic stimuli by reorganising its structure and functions after injury or illness. Where it's a recovery from a stroke or serious brain injury – you are utilising a similar construct. People regain motor control, after a pathway is inhibited and then regrown re forged through persistence. When the onset of a condition changes the way your nervous system flows, You can write new pathways. Rewrite old pathways. Encode new pathways. You can do this by choice by repeatedly using certain techniques. To modify the pathways such that you can control and reduce the sensation of pain where it is chronic. By creating new pathways new learned pathways for the inclusion of intrinsic thought patterns which stimulate the pleasure sensations mimicking orgasm and arousal but subtly, so they are almost undiscernible to the external perspective, that would be a hugely advantageous position.
To integrate a neural pathway for the below sequence – which could be slow or rapid through imagination and repeated visualization dissociated from the elicit sexual image but a simple mental journey, around your own body in your mind, so you can switch on start the sequence, it runs through to completion there is a rush in sensation and a flooding of the nervous system of the hormones oxytocin and dopamine and serotonin and all silent to the outside world.

Imagine "when harry met sally " the famous clip, then imagine a calm confident woman or man simply breathing steadily holding the sensation within, as their central nervous system mentally you run the sequence, almost poker faced, perhaps with the flush of a smile, a relief. A sigh. Very innocuous but great relief.
You choose how you do. You choose.

Because the motive is different.

The motive is what defines the physical pronouncement of expression, so the motive is relief.

And the subtlety is what makes it remarkably possible to

pursue and progress even beyond birthing. The moral. That
the possibilities will go wherever you are prepared to take
them. But they are yours to take. It's all here. Written in
these pages. What is possible. It takes work, it takes everyday
practice, and commitment and belief, when all of these are
aligned, you will see results. There are contraindications like
addiction, and especially where there are cardiac concerns,
but with any thing in life when it's used with balance and a
responsible mind there is the degree of self-control. Common
sense and the interactions you would have with your medical professionals. There are reports of individuals who have
trialled these sequences for (outside of child birth) pain relief.
Who have been mocked or not believed by their medical prac-
titioners. My opinion is if you find a medical practitioner who
works with the mind also, they will be open to the possibility.
There are many. Because they are learning the constructs
of Personal development and adding alternative medicines
and approaches to their practice too. But also, Always always
always, to continue to take your medication and engage any
changes on the advice of your GP (UK) or medical practitioner
overseeing your care and treatment.

Here is just one very basic induction ... you can adapt as you
choose to personalise. You can include self stimulation touch
or any route to amplify the sensation, which effectively is
intended to turn orgasm from a physical experience to mental
experience In this context only, so you can utilise the sensations with alternate purpose and introduce a new facet of
intimacy and correlation with controlling your own sense of
pain. Responsibly. And enjoy a healthy sex life.
Below is one very basic induction. Once again it's very different but in the privacy of your own mind, make it work.

Simply close your eyes and let everything else fade away
in importance. I want you to think of the word relax ......
Think about how it has two syllables Re lax... As you breathe
in think Re to yourself. And as you breathe out Think lax
Don't let your mind wander away for repeating the word relax
When you breathe out try to let go of any tension
in your body

Focus on those muscles, which may have
been holding some tension
Every time you breathe out lax the out
breath is the one to focus on.

The in breath takes care of itself

Think re on each breath in
and lax on each breath out.
Imagine you are on at the edge of a rainforest and
see the effervescence of the light that is above
you reaching through the tree canopy.
All around you is a sense of vibrancy and nourishment
a sense of calm and eternal life within the plants and
the richness of the life that surrounds them, flows
through them and the more you become aware of
it the stronger it becomes it grows and builds like
it they are pulsating with life and vigour.
The vivacity of the space around you simply
begins to become you
as you breathe in, you breathe in you breathe in the
the richness of the eternal life and vigour, ad you
breathe in you breathe in health and as you breathe
out you breathe out any thoughts or fears worries they
just dissolve as you absorb the vivacity of the space
around you within it nourishes you and feeds your
body and mind and the effervescence becomes you,
nourishing relaxing every cell of your body.
Like a breathe of fresh air that fills you with a
sense of calm, the warmth of the air around you is
comforting, it is not too warm and not too cold just
right as you continue to breathe in you continue to
relax and the sense of aliveness consumes you,
you know its ok to let go and relax,
as you breathe in you breathe in calm and as
you breathe out you breathe out tension.
Each breath fulfils you.

And you Reeel aaaax You reee laaaax Calm confident
and in control

Each breath

And you are feeling completely in control
Allow your hands to rest comfortably on top of your
legs wherever they feel most comfortable
Now as you relax more and let it go more and more You can
allow every muscle in your body to relax Every cell every
nerve every fibre in your body relaxing Now picture in your

mind a candle this candle can be any colour you with it to be
The colour you have chosen for your candle is a colour you
unconscious mind knows relaxes you and calms your mind.
Calms you and relaxes your mind. It is your colour of calm,
Now focus on you the colour of the flame of the candle.
See how amazing the colours within the flame are.
You may see red, blue yellow purple white
And maybe another colour.
And as you see the colours within the
flame you relax more and more
And go deeper Keeping the golden hue of the
warmth in your mind as a ball.
A ball of relaxation which will go with you wherever
you choose wherever you direct your attention.
And as you enjoy these heavy and relaxed feelings
deeply relaxed feelings.
These feelings of being in control.
And you continue to see the light of the
warmth of the golden ball.
Now imagine that you re that candle a candle
of relaxation and you are relaxed.
Initially.
Now moving your attention away from the candle begin
to imagine the warmth a like a golden ball of light.
It's as if it's under your skin and working its way through
your body with a glowing comfort and warmth where
ever it touches it expands the sensation of comfort and
arousal, you know you remember the feeling of arousal,
not the place the person because you are the person who
became aroused, bringing the sensation only to mind, the
sensation very softly very subtly but it glows a warm glow
and it feels to a warms glowing warm sensation exciting
the nerves and areas it touches with its warmth, bringing
to life the sensation of pleasure and building in its warmth
and glow pulsating with excitement and enlivenment.
It's easily discernible where it's moving, and it moves with
your attention as you can see it in your mind's eye.
This glowing ball moves as you will it, but it sits
underneath beneath your skin like a layer of comfort a
layer of warmth, without even touching your body you can
control where the energy moves to. It can have a colour.
It brings with it the sensation of warmth a tingling
sensation of arousal, tingling sensation so invisible
touch of pure pleasure.
This invisible touch increases instructs your body to produce

the hormones oxytocin, dopamine, and serotonin they
are all golden and increase as the golden light expands.
As this invisible touch increases these hormones
and expands them with each breath.
Each time you envisage the glowing golden ball
these hormones increase in intensity.
As they do you experience a sensation of a flush of pure
golden light filing your senses with pleasure flushing through
the areas of pain and giving them a momentous flush of
relief. The effervescence of the rainforest glow resembles
the sense of the flush of pure and perfect health which
now surrounds your cells in your mind as you allow the
sensations of pain to dissolve. As you can envision the nerve
endings like the branches of a tree, the branches of a tree filled
with the warm sensation of relief and absolute pleasure.
And it lingers.
Floods and flushes through the sensations of pain with a
powerful golden sense of warmth and you feel a deep sense
comfort, relief, but you can still focus, you can still attend
to your normal daily activities you are simply relaxed,
with a greater sense of relief and can return to the place.
With the candle in your mind's eye at any time should
you choose to awaken the relief once again.
You can even use one simple word to instruct
your mind to begin.
This will be a word very personal to you. And
be used for this specific purpose only.
(state it to your mind quietly now)
You can return at any time to revivify and strengthen this
place, your personal place where you can control your own
pain.
It expands increasing the sensation of arousal very
gently, building and building then it multiplies and send
another glowing golden ball of warmth to your breasts
or nipples, neck, inner thighs, and most intimate places
and other areas (insert your own preferences) then once
the sense of arousal peaks, it moves becomes a ball once
again and mentally you see it move to the exacting place
where your pain once resides. All of the areas are lit with
a gold wave of absolute pleasure building in a warmth not
heat but warmth and tingling as the sensation builds.
Washes a wave of gold warmth through your neurology
expanding with pleasure and expanding with warmth. Flushing through the sensations of pain until they are all but gone.
Until you feel a flush and it so intense that you may just

blush a little and that is ok only as much is as comfortable as
your cells light up with the pleasure sensations expanding
and the sensation of the expansion warmth and arousal
building and expanding the sensation of pleasure like a
flush of colour an expansion almost an explosion of golden
warmth and you reach the pulsating high of orgasmic climax.
Very subtly and very gently.
As you do imagine this golden light filled with
the pleasure hormones oxytocin.
You can adapt this. It can work for the fast climax or
the slow burn and to flood your neurology with a wave
of pleasure hormones. And as you do, you remember
your word. The word than can ignite the pulsation and
experience of the flush of pleasure instantaneously.
You remember this word. Now test it. And flush there is.
You can now turn up the power and amplification of that
sensation, stronger and stronger now. Targeted exactly
where you need it so strong you can see it as a flush of
golden light and a warmth in sensation that excites your
neurology and gives you the sensation of pure pleasure
delivered exactly where you need it to increase the comfort
and have pain sensations subside, be flushed through with
the sensation of pure pleasure. And the purest golden light.

Once again you can imagine a dial to turn up the
intensity of the sensation. Do that now.

And as you do feel the intensity of the sensation increase.

Again remember your chosen word so these sensations can
become instantly available to you as and when you need.

Then by chance you remember the rain forest, and the
pleasant sensation of the vivacity of the canopy above
you, it is so fresh and lush and the air somehow even
more clear with a sense of familiarity now meaning
that you can always return to the place where you were.
Always return to the rainforest canopies to go inside and
reignite your bond with the sensation amplification.

For now though it is time to awaken.

And return to your normal consciousness with a
freshness and vibrance, knowing that something
has changed and that is ok.

9 8 7 6 5 4321 and you are fully alert awake in the room integrated and in harmony with the world around you.
To practice this process until you can simply imagine a golden ball, and intend its location and feel immediate relief.

And it's use beyond birthing is very much a possibility. The most pertinent point within Birthing babies with the Big O is that you have the ability to move your world with your mind, Your body the way it feels, are all influenced by the sequence and quality of your thoughts and intentions. The direction of your experience can be changed on a cellular level by the change in perspective of your beliefs about what is possible especially with the trajectory of pain versus pleasure. The two were born and designed to work concurrently in childbirth so they could work beside each other and give others the strength to birth in a way that is synonymous with conception. The reverberation of the sensation and motive of pleasure in birth, will undulate through each and every cellular interaction between mother and baby so that being born becomes a time of great excitement without fear.
Be kind to yourself.
Imagining the comparison and the moment a child enters this world, even when the environment is forced clinical nature you can still control the sensations in your body and your mind, and you can still desensitise the sensations of fear so that birth even with intervention is a very positive experience for you and your baby. You can. You can because you are more than you thought you were. You have a different perspective that shows you what you are capable of. In doing this you increase the sensations of physical health and well and your ability to heal. Overcoming the incumbencies to the healing process which would be resembled and represented by the heavier negative emotions such as fear and guilt, these are overcome by knowing you are doing everything in your power to make your birthing expense one of choice and one of pleasure for both you and a baby. And of the practices included in birthing babies and birthing babies with the big O are relevant in contributing to this layer by layer.

Through this book you have learned .... Each one in your mind can form a layer, a new layer of strength of belief a of internal support. A layer of confidence a layer of competence and with each layer you begin to build. Within you are stronger and more able because that is what knowledge does, compound by belief.

Compound is to strengthen, it is how coal turns to diamond. Repeat. repeat. repeat. You won't even notice them building but you will notice them at a point in the future when you reflect and notice things have changed.

You will take a retrospective glance six twelve months in to the future and look back and notice.

How far you have come, how much you have achieved and how much stronger you are, how much more confident and how you can review your birthing experience as a positive experience.

Building your ability to manage your own experience of pain, and how effective that can be.

Because you formed the layers. Without even thinking. It takes commitment to reading to listening and to practicing. To using the guided visualisations.

So all it leaves is for you to do, to use what you have read, integrated and learned, to experiment, to learn your body so it is there when you need it the.

Most, to build a confidence in your body, to expand your self acceptance, becoming more sexually adept in a way that is complementary to you as a woman and strengthens your feminine resolve. That is within your parameters of acceptance and so is defined by you as to what is acceptable.

You are the leader, you choose. Embrace the Big O and make it your own. But without compromise. Make it right for you.

Now you know, The cycle of arousal. What an orgasm is the stages how to make the, how to harness them, The female sexual body. So now you know, and can identify What an orgasm is, The stages of orgasm, The layers and how they can translate into the stages of child birth and it actually makes sense when it is overlayed.

Thy types of orgasm, an introduction to your body, and the places you can make excite to make that happen and how to make them happen.

Your uterus Its intricate structure and the emerging purpose for the orgasmic template.

The stages of labour and what it means to overlay the orgasmic template, through your birthing experience. The chemical sequences, how to orchestrate the synergy of your dynamic organic structures and sequences, and how it makes sense so you can use it. You are familiar with your uterus, its role function and form and your erogenous zones, places to try places to learn and places to love.

You know the intricate structure of your uterus, The pain pleasure paradigm, how to reverse pain sensations, how to breathe to pervade calm, the mind body connection, the purity of the origination of your physical makeup on. A cellular level and how to influence this with each act thought word and deed. The construction, production and mixture of biochemical synergy that occurs in labour and orgasm, the orgasmic template overlaying birth.

The process and progress of labour, what will happen how it will feel and what to do when it does, you know how to control your energy and focus when birthing, how to move your body and position for ease. To overlay the orgasmic template in labour step by step at your very own pace. When and how to move your body in synergy with the flow of labour, for efficiency and comfort.
The divergence of carnal desire and overlaying the orgasmic template in birth. Acceptance of the feminine and your ability to bridge the divide in religious social and cultural beliefs and condescension. How to bridge the cultural and generational divide mentally so you can find acceptance that overlaying the orgasmic template is acceptable. The definition of the space of union in the feminine and encouragement to embrace the contrast in life. The importance and essentials for intimacy and how they are mirrored in birth. The ability to communicate with your midwife, introduce the concept. And pertinently how to expand the potential for the orgasmic template to all forms of chronic pain moving forwards. The journey begins through pregnancy exploring the deepest aspects of your sexual nature, The woman who is everything can really begin to be everything. Overcome challenges through pregnancy and labour and begin to enjoy a new acceptance of her own sensuality and birth. To enjoy the process of engaging with relaxation techniques.
You now have choice confidence and are able to assert your choices with grace and confidence.

To explore parts of your self that were previously dormant. Of your body you did not even conceive of in the past. To build a beautiful synergy with your self as a confident woman, a mother, a lover and a woman who births. Replacing pain with pleasure. Bringing together harmony within your body in birth, to form new and meaningful associations and bring great joy to your life in all ways.

Cosmic!

IMPORTANT NOTE.

*There are contraindications for everything and
here is the reminder for birthing babies.*

*The materials in Victoria Whitney's books are provided on an as
is basis.
For the purposes of education and entertainment.*

*Victoria Whitney makes no warranties expressed or implied
and hereby disclaims and negates all other warranties included
within content, online courses trainings, including without
limitation. Implied warranties or conditions of merchantability
fitness for a particular purpose or non infringement of
intellectual property, contestation of service delivery as described
or other violation of rights*

*Further victoria Whitney does not warrant or make any
representation concerning the accuracy likely of results
or reliability of the use of terms on consultation or
materials on its books or programs of guidance used in
sessions and recommended or otherwise such relating to
the to the materials on this site and session content.*

*Consult your doctor if you have an underlying health
condition, Heart condition or any other underlying health
condition before you undertake any of the above activities.*

It's not recommended for people who:

- *have had a prior C-section*

- *are pregnant with multiples*

- *have certain health conditions*

Without seeking medical advice. It is important to Discuss with your doctor any health concerns you have before undertaking any form of new health regimen.

cluding the right to reproduce this book or portions thereof, in any form. No part of this text may be reproduced in any form without the express written permission of the author.

The publisher and the author strongly recommend that you consult with your physician before beginning any exercise program. You should be in good physical condition and be able to participate in the exercises expressed within this book. The author is not a licensed healthcare care provider and represents that they have no expertise in diagnosing, examining, or treating medical conditions of any kind, or in determining the effect of any specific exercise on a medical condition.

You should understand that at any time during labour you could require the assistance of medical professional.

Always seek medical advice if you are concerned. The author and publisher accepts no responsibility or liability for your failure to do so, OR any representative damage, personal, physical or otherwise, or loss which could occur as a result from the omission to do so.

If you engage in these activities Scripts and guidance does not replace the requirement for professional medical advice. In reading this book and using these practices you, you agree that you do so at your own risk, are voluntarily participating in these activities, assume all risk of injury to yourself, and agree to release and discharge the publisher and the author from any and all claims or causes of action, known or unknown, arising out of the contents of this book.

The publisher and the author advise you to take full responsibility for your safety and know your limits. Before practicing the skills described in this book, be sure that your equipment is well maintained and do not take risks beyond your level of experience, aptitude, training, Condition of health and mind and comfort level.

Although the publisher and the author have made every effort to ensure that the information in this book was correct at press time and while this publication is designed to provide accurate information in regard to the subject matter covered, the publisher and the author assume no responsibility for errors, inaccuracies, omissions, or any other inconsistencies herein and hereby disclaim any liability to any party for any loss, damage, or disruption caused by errors or omissions, whether such errors or omissions result from negligence, accident, or any other cause.

Unless otherwise indicated, all the names, characters, businesses, places, events and incidents in this book are either the product of the author's imagination or used in a fictitious manner. Any resemblance to actual persons, living or dead, or actual events is purely coincidental.

The publisher and the author make no guarantees concerning the level of success you may experience by following the advice and strategies contained in this book, and you accept the risk that results will differ for each individual. The testimonials and examples provided in this book show exceptional results, which may not apply to the average reader, and are not intended to represent or guarantee that you will achieve the same or similar results.

This book is not intended as a substitute for the medical advice of physicians. The reader should regularly consult a physician in matters relating to their health, particularly with respect to any symptoms that may require diagnosis or medical attention.

Cover Illustration Copyright © 2026 by Victoria Whitney

Cover design by Victoria Whitney

Book design and production by Victoria Whitney

Editing by Victoria Whitney

Chapter opening illustrations all illustrations © 2026 Victoria Whitney

Simply close you eyes and let everything
else fade away in importance

I want you to think of the word relax ......

Think about how it has two syllables

Re lax......

As you breathe in think

Re to yourself

And as you breathe out

Think lax

Don't let your mind wander away for repeating the word relax

When you breathe out try to let go of any tension
in your body

Focus on those muscles, which may have
been holding some tension

Every time you breathe out lax the out
breath is the one to focus on

The in breath takes care of itself

Think re on each breath in and lax on each breath out

Imagine those out breaths

Are being blown into a big balloon all of your
tensions being expelled from your body and
being blown into that big balloon

The balloon being filled up with air and when
it is full imagine it floating away

And as it floats away the balloon carries
away all of those tensions

And you are feeling completely in control

Allow your hands to rest comfortably on top of your
legs wherever they feel most comfortable

Now as you relax more and let it go ore and more

You can allow every muscle in your body to relax

Every cell every nerve every fiber in your body relaxing

Now picture in your mind a candle this candle
can be any color you with it to be

The color you have chosen for your candle is a color you
unconscious mind knows relaxes you and calms your mind

Calms you and relaxes your mind. It is your color of calm

Now focus on you the color of the flame of the candle

See how amazing the colors within the flame are

You may see red, blue yellow purple white

And maybe another color

And as you see the colors within the flame
you relax more and more

And go deeper

And as you enjoy these heavy and relaxed feelings
deeply relaxed feelings

These feelings of being in control.

Now focus on the wax body of your candle

Now see the first trickle of melting wax
begin to move down the wax

Now see the melting wax touch the candleholder and
merge with it to become part of the candleholder

You become more and more relaxed

Feeling safe and comfortable

Now imagine that you re that candle

A candle of total relaxation

And as you picture it a particular muscle in
your body melts away its tension allowing you
to relax more and more completely

Picture whatever you are sitting or lying on as a candle holder
and that you re becoming yourself a candle of relaxation

Feel yourself melting into the experience of childbirth

Your body simply melting into the task of
doing what it knows how to do

You are feeling calm confident and in control

And because you are feeling calm confident and in control

your body follows your mind as your mind relaxes

And your mind follows your body

As our body relaxes

Your baby too is feeling calm trusting the experience
and trusting you

Notice how you have to bee n aware of any sensations of
the area of your body that your hands have been resting
on until you choose to switch your awareness there

In the same way you can choose which sensations which
sensations to be aware of or to focus on during you labor

Now I will count form 1 up to 10

And as I count I want you to imagine you are seeing
your baby for the first time

1, 2, 3,

Notice how much more in control you are feeling

Four

Five

Calm confident and in control

6

7

8

Becoming more aware of the room now

9

Because you choose to become aware of the room

10

In your own time open your eyes and become aware of the room

GUIDED RELAXATION SESSION 2

ALLOW YOUR EYES TO GENTLY CLOSE

Just let the outside world simply fade away

Give your thoughts time to become still and quiet

Notice whatever sound you can hear around you

Maybe the sounds of the music in the back ground

Maybe the gently ticking of a clock

Maybe even the sound of the air moving within the room

Be aware of the sound of your own breathing

Allow these sounds to become part

Of your experience

Allow them to become more important to you

Imagine that there is a little person inside your mind

And that little person is sweeping up all of the worries the cares

The words

The thoughts and the concerns of the day

Gently blow the dust away in the quietness and the stillness
that is left imagine that you re at the beginning of your labour
its now time for your baby to be born

Nothing is expected of you

There is nothing you have to do

You don't even have to listen to my voice

You don't need to do anything but to enjoy the feelings that come

To enjoy the feelings f relaxation that increase with every breath you take

And increasing with each word that I speak

Gently focus into your breathing

Notice the gentle rise and fall of your chest

With each easy breath

Imagining breathing the calmness

And breathing out the tension

Breathing in calmness

And breathing out tension

Just like a sigh

If calmness had a colour

Imagine what that colour would be for you

What would the colour of calm be for you

See it

Sense it

Feel it

Imagine yourself surrounded by that colour of calm just
like a warm swirling soothing mist of calm each tie you
breathe in you are breathing in that colour of calm

If tension had a colour

Imagine what that colour would be

What would the colour of tension be for you

See it sense it

Feel it

Imagine breathing out that t colour of tension

As you are breathing in that colour of calmness

Breathing out the colour of tension

Breathing in calmness

And breathing out tension

Just like a sigh

Find your own natural rhythm feel those breaths in reaching
right down to your baby

Soothing your baby

Sending positive messages to your baby

That everything is well

Acting like a very soothing anaesthetic

Breathing yourself down into peacefulness

Down into calm ness

Down into stillness of mind

Experience your body reacting to this deep relaxation

Imagine that you are standing in a beautiful path of rain forest

This lush rainforest runs along by a beautiful stretch of sandy beach

You have been walking through the resin forest in the direction of the each

The last bit of inclined forest path

This lush rain forest runs along a beautiful stretch of sandy

beach you have been walking through the rain forest in the
direction of the beach the last bit of inclined forest path will
eventually lead you out into the sandy shores of the beach

But before you leave the rain forest you stop and stand

And look above and take in the lush greens and take in the canopy of the lush
rain forest trees you can see the strong sunlight beaming through the foliage

Like rays of glistening energy

You can hear exotic birds

And sounds that soothe you with a reminder that nature
s happening all around

The smell of the air is crisp clean and fresh and
alive with wonderful exotic smells

The birds are singing so happily and chattering to other birds in the forest

You take-in a few deep breaths to smell the abundant rain forest aromas

And as you breathe out

Relax - deeper and deeper

And as you continue on your way

You come to a winding pathway which leads you out of a

Down onto the beach

It may be one which is familiar to you

Or one which you have constructed in your imagination

Notice how eager you are to descent to the beach

The sand

Looks golden and inviting

And as you descend

I will count from ten down to one

And you will be standing on the beach

Start descending down onto the beach

Ten

Nine

You are getting closer to your beach

Eight

Seven

You are feeling more

Six

Five

More an more relaxed

Four almost there

Three

Two

You are now standing on the beach feeling very relaxed and happy

The beach is everything you dreamed it to be

Stretching out before you is miles of incredible white golden sand

As you slowly walk along relaxing deeper and deeper with each step

Notice what you re wearing

You are feeling confident

And comfortable

As you slip of your shoes stretch and stroll across the gold
sand you feel the warm sand under the soles of your feet
you can see the grains glistening in the sunlight

There is no one but you here

Simply enjoying some precious time to yourself

You stand and marvel at the incredible view

The brilliant mixes of jade green and iridescent views of the ocean foreshore

You gaze out into the distance of the calm blue sea

And see the vastness stretching out before you

Marvelling at the spaciousness and the sense of freedom

There is a fishing boat in the distance with its colourful sail

Gently bobbing up and down

The sun is shining

The sky is blue

And not a cloud in sight

Take a moment to notice what gentle sound you can hear

Perhaps there are some seagulls in the distance

Perhaps you can hear the peaceful a lapping of the waves

Perhaps you can hear your own gentle breathing

Perhaps you can hear your own

Take a few moments to notice hat else you an hear

You are embarking on one of the most incredible experiences of your life

you are feeling so relaxed and your whole body feels comfortably
loose and limp and relaxed

You hear the sounds of the leaves and your whole body feels relaxed

The breeze keeps your face cool and the sun continues
to energise your whole body

And you watch how the waves roll towards the beach

In a never ending sequence one after another and
then petering out as they near the beach

You walk towards the waters edge

Witnessing the immense power of nature enabling the waves
to move forward before receding into the wet sand

And when you reach the sea you gently let your toes test the water

Which is slightly cool as you take few more steps into the
water you are feeling the immense power of nature

A normal natural process

And as you allow the waves to roll over your feet and ankles and retreat again

You breathe in the salty sea air and relax deeper and deeper

As you allow the waves to roll over your feet and
ankles and then retreat again

You breathe in the fresh salty sea air

And relax deeper.

You realize that just like the surging of the waves is a process you can see
and feel so what is happening in your body is a normal natural process

A physiological process that your body knows how to do

You walk as far as the small waves

Where you let your feet feel the cool washes of the
water the water washes over your ankles

They roll in like delicate rushes of energy

As the waves within your own body become more powerful

It is a constant reminder that you an trust your body

I trust my body it knows what to do

You feel a growing feeling of peace and calm

As the warm sea air lightly brushes your skin

And as your feet sink into the sand beneath the
water with every step you take

So you are relaxing deeper and deeper with each step

And you notice much the sea is up close

As wave after wave rolls up towards you

Each contraction will bring me closer towards the birth of my baby

Each contraction has its own job to do

Once that contraction has gone I will never be able to experience
that contraction again

Each contraction in your body

Each one a reminder that your body knows what to do

I trust my body it knows what to do

Labour is a normal

Physiological process

The natural moments of the waves remind you of the a natural
movements within your body

As you notice a contraction within your body

You tilt your head slightly upwards towards the sun

You feel the suns energy and light al over your face

It feels like the sun its there for you and for no one else

The feeling brings a small smile to your face

And you instinctively know all is well within your body and with your baby

Nothing in the world is bothering you now

Any small worries or anxieties leave your mind as they surface –

Watch them drift out to sea

On the gentle breeze after a while you stroll back up the beach to
a most inviting deck chair which sit there especially for you

And there is a sunshade and a table

And your favourite refreshing drink

And as you adjust the sunshade so its just right for you

As you lies back in the chair and you relax deeper
and deeper still and you breathe out

When you need hydration your body send clear messages
to drink water to refresh and revitalize you

When you need something more for your baby your body will send
a clear and comfortable sign to look towards a professional

While sitting there identify any worries you have at this time about labour
about child birth and parent hood imagine them leaving your mind and
coming back as learnings , integrations or solutions and new options

As they float away on the wind out to sea telling yourself the
worries have now gone as you lie there on the warm sand
with the sea breezes washing over your face you notice your
breathing has slowed down to a comfortable pace
The solutions the faith, the direction and the confidence remain.

Your breaths are less frequent

Your whole body is safe warm and

Your mind is calm

You are at peace

I trust my body

It knows what to do

And because you are so calm our body will be free to progress
your labour and your baby will be calm also

For now enjoy the sea breezes and enjoy the warmth of the sun

Spend as long as you want on your beach before taking three deep breaths
and exhaling fully before starting to breathe at your usual rate again

Wriggle your fingers and your toes

This will help your mind to renter your body

And when you feel ready

Slowly open your eyes

And take a few moments to enjoy the calm and relaxed feelings
that now linger over you

And notice your environment and the people around you

Retaining that sense of calm and knowing that you can return to your
beach by counting down from ten to one whenever it feels right to do so

This incredible experience is just short way into the future
leaving you some time to visit your beach

Building up anticipation and excitement about this time with your baby

But for now

I am going to count

From one

To ten

And as I do you will feel more and more alert

More and more refreshed

Confident in the knowledge that you can do this

A renewed faith in yourself and your body

One

Two
three
four
five
six
seven
eight
nine
ten

Simply close your eyes and let everything
else fade away in importance

I want you to think of the word relax ......

Think about how it has two syllables

Re lax...

As you breathe in think

Re to yourself

And as you breathe out

Think lax

Don't let your mind wander away for repeating the word relax

When you breathe out try to let go of any tension
in your body

Focus on those muscles, which may have
been holding some tension

Every time you breathe out lax the out
breath is the one to focus on

The in breath takes care of itself

Think re on each breath in and lax on each breath out

Imagine those out breaths

Are being blown into a big balloon all of your
tensions being expelled from your body and
being blown into that big balloon

The balloon being filled up with air and when
it is full imagine it floating away

And as it floats away the balloon carries
away all of those tensions

And you Reeel aaaax You reee laaaax

Calm confident and in control

Each breath

And you are feeling completely in control

Allow your hands to rest comfortably on top of your
legs wherever they feel most comfortable

Now as you relax more and let it go ore and more

You can allow every muscle in your body to relax

Every cell every nerve every fiber in your body relaxing

Now picture in your mind a candle tis candle
can be any color you with it to be

The color you have chose n for your candle is a color you
unconscious mind knows relaxes you and calms your mind

Calms you and relaxes your mind. It is your color of calm

Now focus on you the color of the flame of the candle

See how amazing the colors within the flame are

You may see red, blue yellow purple white

And maybe another color

And as you see the colors within the flame
you relax more and more

And go deeper

And as you enjoy these heavy and relaxed feelings
deeply relaxed feelings

These feelings of being in control.

Now focus on the wax body of your candle

Now see the first trickle of melting wax
begin to move down the wax

Now see the melting wax touch the candleholder and
merge with it to become part of the candleholder

You become more and more relaxed

Feeling safe and comfortable

Now imagine that you re that candle

A candle of total relaxation

Now within this relaxation you can think towards
a safe place inside

Within that safe place you will have a space to
build an experience of the unknown.

You can imagine now that you are within the preparation
for your theatre you are prepared and feeling calm confident
and in control your re surrounded by professionals
who know what to do to help you birth your baby

So you can be calm confident and in control

The room smells clinical and that's of comfort, as you
know it's a safe way to right baby on this day

The sounds the colors you can acclimatize very quickly

You remember the candle the candle of ultimate relaxation

Any nerves or fears can simply dissolve as you have
a sense of comfort and priority to bright baby with
ease faith love and safely maintaining that sense
of comfort always knowing that you are doing the

right thing for you and the right thing for baby

And you remember the candle the candle of ultimate
relaxation and feel calm confident and in control

The sense of the room is professional and clean though
you have the sense of growing warmth and love within
you building and building and feeling of greater comfort

You move towards the theater and as you go though the
doors you can small the clean and fresh environment
you can sense the setting is ok, its safe and you feel
comfortable to proceed with the procedure

As you prepare you may be required to lie down or sit upon
the edge of the bed for a small numbing treatment. It feels
totally normal. It feels totally comfortable. You know what
to expect. You are calm confident and in control any fears or
worries can just release as you breathe in calm and breathe
out tension breathe in calm and breathe out tension

As you do you feel calm confident and strong within

Each moment is taking you closer to birthing your baby safely

Each and every breath you take is bringing you
closer to birthing your baby so you enter into
the theatre and you lie on the table

The clothes and gowns and masks feel appropriate and
you have a growing sense of comfort knowing that each
moment is bringing you closer to birthing your baby

You can hear the instruments whirring in the background
and the lights are bright, but that is ok as you already knew
that was going to happen and that feels comfortable

You have a sense of warmth and comfort within
you through you and around you and a strong sense
also to enjoy the experience of birthing baby

To be aware and to be alive and to feel the comfortable
sense of calm confident awareness growing within you

As you look up and see the gowns and the doctors at their
work you may hear the tinkling of the medical instruments
in the room and each moment and each sound that you
recognize gives you a deepening sense of comfort and
sense of control within that comfort knowing that each
breath and each moment that passes is bringing you
closer to birthing your baby as time passes the surgeons
may speak with you and update you they will guide you
so you know what is happening moment by moment

And the sense of comfort within you remains
strong with each breath in.

As you take one now and relax knowing that everything is ok

And you remember the candle the candle of ultimate
relaxation and feel calm confident and in control

As you hear the sound of the tinkling instruments
and you may feel sense of pressure under
your ribs just before baby is born

As you do you breathe in and relax and allow the
process to continue knowing that each moment and
each breath brings you closer to birthing your baby

Any discomfort you can remember the candle within and the
dials the internal dials to switch down the discomfort once
its message has been heard you can turn the dials down

Then you can hear the sound of your baby's cry as you
imagine looking up and baby is there. So your body can
now begin to synthesize the hormone oxytocin the love
drug because it can and it can increase the sense of love
and healing for your body and for bonding with t baby.
The moment you hear baby's cry's and see baby your
body responds to the birth with the production of the
love hormone so you can accelerate your physical healing
and form bond with baby and move through the coming
hours days and weeks with a strong sense of love bonding
with baby feeding baby and bonding with baby

And you remember the candle the candle of ultimate
relaxation and feel calm confident and in control as you see
the candle in your minds eye you know your body is healing
and using it energy and nutrients to birth you and baby

Your body can heal and is healing every breath
you now take without conscious thought or
effort you are now healing renewing

Bond with a baby and feel baby on your skin your body's
natural response immediately as baby bonds with you bond
with baby and feel that deepening sense of strength and
comfort as you progress the sense of comfort you have is
deepening and beginning fill your whole body that sense of
great love and joy combined as the relief that baby is here

There resting on your chest

You can smell them and feel their tiny arms and
legs moving now outside of your body and the
beauty of the experience is all encompassing

The love with you and baby and that moment will be within
you for the whole of your life together and always be safe
and protected in your mind and remembered when needed
so you can stay calm confident and in control if you ever
experience a sense of unease or not enough ness you can
remember that bond that strength that love and that love
will move you forward to make the very best things happen .

And you take a deep breath in and this memory begins
to fade but its fades into moments and seconds of
your future time and living memory so it becomes to
the future so you can stay firmly present in the now
and enjoy each moment of life throughout.

And as you do you can remaining very relaxed take
a few moments to breathe in and out and in

And out and then as I count form one to 10 on the
number ten you will awaken alert and in the room.

One

Two

Three

Four

Five

Six

Seven

Eight

Nine

Ten

calming fears.

There is a point of origin, of the fears you experience,
which is so simple, so small, and it was decided, observed
and imprinted long ago when you didnt know any
different, The benefit of the ow is that you can know
you can decide and you can choose to learn from what
you have evolved to know now through time back to
the point you decided to fear it and bring comfort faith
and confidence through all of those memories.

Similar with Anger, frustration, sadness and hurt, even
guilt. The below sequence is effective with each. in turn.

First – The Illusion of time Journey through
the doorways to the sands of Time.

Relax take a deep breath

And another deep breath

Beach, on the beach Imagine a Door way, a door
way to the sands of time, to the sands of time

You open the door, You walk through the open door,
and feel your feet crossing the threshold.

Through the door and its dark inside. But you can see
a light inside, as you look towards the light inside.

As you become aware of the sights and sounds the
sensations of the beach, and the sands of time.

You become aware of a path, a pathway across the
beach it can be in any direction you wish, you make it
so, this is the same form as your life, the line that passes
through now and has a beginning and an end,

Imaging your life time as if it has a beginning and
an end a line of time that has a Past and a future
- This is your life time or time line.

Float up above this line, so you are looking down at
the beach and the pathway below, always staying
above so high so high peaceful up here

Float over your past life time line to the space directly above
the origin of the fears, the decision, the place where origins
of the doubt origins of the beliefs that aren't supportive,
where you didn't believe you could be a mother that it wasn't
easy to birth your baby safely calmly comfortably and
confidently. Always staying ABOVE the line looking down.

Above your life time above the event what did you
need to learn what did you need to know such that
if you had know in it would have been ok

What did you need to learn as you observe those
learnings knowing you have everything you
need inside to let the fears and old beliefs

Those learnings will be retained by your unconscious mind
and stay within you working for you forever whenever you
need them they will be there bringing faith and confidence

Float to the place before the event or any of the events
that led to the event way up high so high above and
notice the old decisions and beliefs have disappeared

Thats right notice inside how it feels very different
now. What is there instead... the feelings notice

how you feelings have changed.

As you float now down into the event notice how
it feel different now. That's right its changed

If there's anything left float back up to before the
event happened and notice the one extra learning
you didn't get that now you have it the negative
emotions and decisions have disappeared.

Now float back to now above that line as quickly as
you can revisit each subsequent event re-evaluate it
in the light of the new choices you have made

As you do notice at least three incidences where
you could have decided differently and know
you have and how different is now.

Then float down into the room. Look around and
notice how it feels different now. How many ways
you can see that things have changed.

Now imagine a time in the past you used to feel those
old fears and notice how it feels differently now

Imagine a time in the future where you used to experience
these old beliefs and notice how it feel differently now.

And then notice how many ways your feelings have changed.

ACKNOWLEDGEMENT

references

1. (Arms, 1994) .https://www.britishjournalofmidwifery.com/content/literature-review/pain-and-pleasure-in-the-birthing-room-understanding-the-phenomenon-of-orgasmic-birth/#B2

2. Davis E, Pascali-Bonaro D. Orgasmic birth your guide to a safe, satisfying and pleasurable birth experience.New York: Rodale; 2010

3.   https://www.britishjournalofmidwifery.com/content/literature-review/pain-and-pleasure-in-the-birthing-room-understanding-the-phenomenon-of-orgasmic-birth/#B8

4. Childbirth climax: the revealing of obstetrical orgasm. 2013. https://www.em-consulte.com/en/article/849520

5. Khajehei M, Doherty M. Childbirth in pleasure and ecstasy: a fountain of hormones and chemicals. Int J of Childbirth Educ. 2012; 27:(3)73-80 Arms S. Immaculate deception II, myth, magic and birth.Berkeley: Celestial Art; 1994

6. Baird, Wilson, Bladin, Saling, & Reutens, 2004; McKenna, 1999; Swanson & Petrovich, 1998).

7. https://victoria-s-school-f8ca.thinkific.com/ or

http://www.victoriawhitney.com/ click tab: online courses.

8. https://www.britishjournalofmidwifery.com/content/literature-review/pain-and-pleasure-in-the-birthing-room-understanding-the-phenomenon-of-orgasmic-birth/#B9

9. https://victoria-s-school-f8ca.thinkific.com/

10. https://www.britishjournalofmidwifery.com/content/literature-review/pain-and-pleasure-in-the-birthing-room-understanding-the-phenomenon-of-orgasmic-birth/#B1

11. https://www.britishjournalofmidwifery.com/content/literature-review/pain-and-pleasure-in-the-birthing-room-understanding-the-phenomenon-of-orgasmic-birth/#B20

12. https://www.britishjournalofmidwifery.com/content/literature-review/pain-and-pleasure-in-the-birthing-room-understanding-the-phenomenon-of-orgasmic-birth/#B8

13. https://www.britishjournalofmidwifery.com/content/literature-review/pain-and-pleasure-in-the-birthing-room-understanding-the-phenomenon-of-orgasmic-birth/#B17

14. https://www.britishjournalofmidwifery.com/content/literature-review/pain-and-pleasure-in-the-birthing-room-understanding-the-phenomenon-of-orgasmic-birth/#B10

15. https://pubmed.ncbi.nlm.nih.gov/4000685/

https://pubmed.ncbi.nlm.nih.gov/22375640/

https://pubmed.ncbi.nlm.nih.gov/26578553/

There are contraindications for everything and here is the reminder for birthing babies Consult your doctor if you have an underlying health condition, Heart condition or any underlying health condition before you undertake any of the above activities. Birthing babies Victoria Whitney disclaim any liability for actions taken by readers as a result of reading this book.

Nor do they abdicate any one path for all. It's not recommended for people who:

- *have had a prior C-section*

- *are pregnant with multiples*

- *have certain health conditions*

It is important to Discuss with your doctor any health concerns you have.

Always seek advice from a medical practitioner before engaging in any alternative health routine. Check with your GP midwife or medical practitioner before engaging in any form of exertion or activity.

This book is for the purposes of advice and entertainment. Readers engage in any of the activities at their own risk.

ABOUT THE AUTHOR

Victoria Whitney

Victoria has a successful career working with 1:1 clients and has also worked in the NHS and Health and social care environment since 2004.

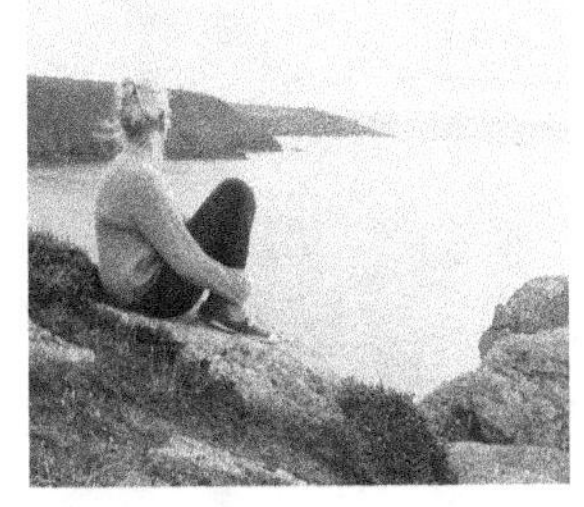

She is the person who can solve any problem, when approached in person. The coaches coach and the go to in her areas of Expertise.

In person she has a wealth and calm essence in addition to her wealth of experience the vibrancy and energy she has are unique.

Victoria is a Multi Award Winning Personal Empowerment Expert Awarded for Inspiring Human Potential and Three times the Winner of the Coach of the Year in the South West of England in 2023 – 2024 2024 – 2025 and 2025 to 2026

With 24 years experience having qualified in Hypnotherapy specifically for child birth in 2012 ahead of the birth of her son. Victoria has a fascinating insightful dynamic which she is renowned for making the most complex of ideas appear very simple. She is so Highly designated in her fields she has won multiple awards. As her ability to balance questions of the Metaphysical realm balanced with her intellectual and insane problem-solving ability is Unrivalled in her Field. She is the Coaches coach. Who the leading experts "go to" to find resolutions. With a successful career in coaching both personal and professional development field.

BOOKS IN THIS SERIES

Birthing Babies

Birthing Babies.
A series built to move you through child birth and into parenthood, with confidence and Empowerment.
Increasing confidence to have a natural birth and true Empowerment for women to make confident educated choices about how they birth.

Birthing Babies- The Ultimate Guide To A Positively Empowered Birth

This is a valuable guide to using Simple techniques, to birth your baby with confidence, Building a deep sense of calm, confidence and in control, centred and Empowered on your journey into and through Motherhood.

Victoria is an Award Winning Personal Empowerment Expert with 21 years experience having qualified in Hypnotherapy specifically for child birth in 2012 ahead of the birth of her son. Victoria has a fascinating insightful dynamic which she is renowned for making the most complex of ideas appear very simple.

Alongside powerful mind set techniques and inspiring motivational perspectives, birthing babies contains fascinating insights into your physical body its makeup and its evolution. Hypnotherapy for child birth as empowering as possible, simple as possible, as accessible as possible right now. The best should be available and accessible to everyone.

The Ultimate Guide to a Positively Empowered Birth brings revelatory insights which give the reader the ability to birth baby with confidence and create a life beyond birth that is synonymous with the greatest vision they have for their future life.

Including :
Your body - Fascinating insights The science of birth made simple (your uterus has never been this sexy)
The birth of confidence - Turning fears into faith
Laboring with love - The transition through the stages of labour simplified guides How your body and baby work together to make this possible
Ultimate positioning -
Postpartum promise - Living the life you wanted.

Full of inspiring and relatable truths to partner and guide you on your road to motherhood and fill you with the ability to confidently enjoy the path through planning, pregnancy birth and beyond.